National League for Nursing



# THE SCOPE OF PRACTICE

## FOR ACADEMIC NURSE EDUCATORS PRACTICING IN VARIOUS ACADEMIC NURSE EDUCATOR ROLES:

### THE FULL SCOPE OF THE EDUCATOR ROLE, THE CLINICAL EDUCATOR ROLE, THE NOVICE EDUCATOR ROLE, AND THE PRACTICAL/ VOCATIONAL EDUCATOR ROLE

*4th Edition*

*Editors*

**Linda S. Christensen, EdD, JD, RN, CNE, FAAN**

**Larry E. Simmons, PhD, RN, CNE, ICE-CCP, CGNC, FAAN**

Wolters Kluwer

Philadelphia • Baltimore • New York • London
Buenos Aires • Hong Kong • Sydney • Tokyo

*Acquisitions Editor:* Heather Bays-Petrovic
*Senior Development Editor:* Staci Wolfson
*Marketing Manager:* Amy Whitaker
*Production Project Manager:* Jennifer L. Harper
*Manager, Graphic Arts & Design:* Stephen Druding
*Manufacturing Coordinator:* Margie Orzech-Zeranko
*Prepress Vendor:* Aptara, Inc.



First printing 2005. Revised 2012. Revised 2020. Revised 2026.

Christensen, L. S., & Simmons, L. E. (2027). *The scope of practice for academic nurse educators practicing in various academic nurse educator roles* (4th ed.). National League for Nursing.



9 8 7 6 5 4 3 2 1

Printed in the United States of America

---

Cataloging in Publication data available on request from publisher.
ISBN-13: 978-1-9752-8216-5

---



shop.lww.com     www.NLN.com

MPP1125

# About the Editors

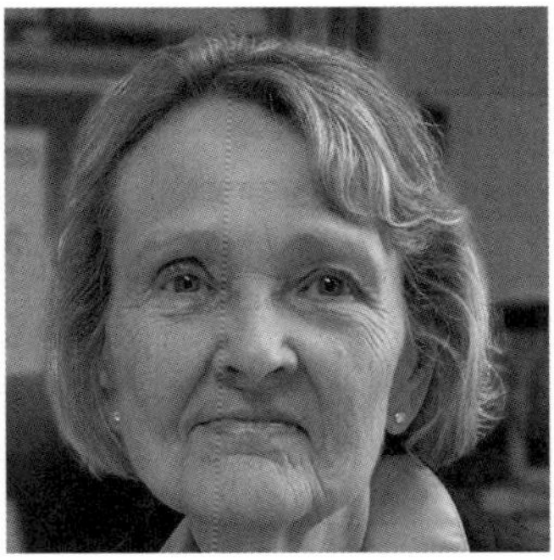

**Linda S. Christensen, EdD, JD, RN, CNE, FAAN**, is chief legal officer for the National League for Nursing and has been with the National League for Nursing for the past 16 years. Her work at the National League for Nursing has included administrative oversight of the Academic Nurse Educator Certification Program, where she has assisted with program administration and new certification program development. She has over 40 years of experience in nursing education, with expertise in nursing education administration, nursing program development, curriculum development, and evaluation. She has taught both graduate and undergraduate nursing, both on campus and online. Additionally, she is an attorney with 25 years of experience in combining nursing and the law. She is a guest speaker on legal issues in nursing education and has authored multiple chapters on nursing law for various nursing education books.

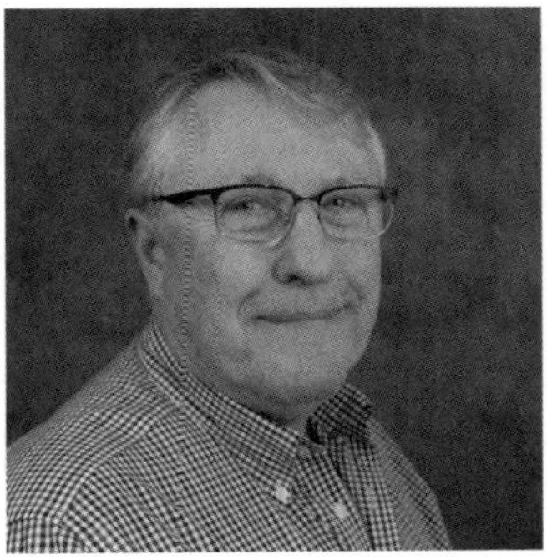

**Larry E. Simmons, PhD, RN, CNE, ICE-CCP, CGNC, FAAN**, is the senior director of the Credentialing Department at the National League for Nursing (NLN). He received an associate's degree in nursing from Metropolitan Community College, a bachelor's degree from the University of Missouri–Kansas City, as well as a master's in nursing and his doctorate degrees. Dr. Simmons is widely known for his expertise in nursing education and in standardized testing, along with the psychometrics of testing results. He has been a nurse educator for more than 20 years, as well as serving as a consultant to many programs of nursing across the United States. He also has a special interest in the global community of nursing education, traveling internationally to promote certification for nurse educators. He has been active in many professional nursing organizations, including the American Assembly of Men in Nursing and Sigma Theta Tau, International. Representing the certification program at NLN, he is also involved in the American Board of Nursing Specialties group.

# Contents

1

# The Development of the Scope of Practice for Academic Nurse Educators Practicing in Various Academic Nurse Educator Roles

## INTRODUCTION

The purpose of this chapter is to describe academic nursing education and academic clinical nursing education as specialty areas and advanced practice nursing roles within professional nursing. The historical perspective, values and beliefs, and theoretical framework of the academic nurse educator role(s), as well as research in these role(s) and the future for the academic nurse educator roles, are presented. Additionally, the discussion of each role includes definitions, scope of practice, standards of practice, and core competencies.

*The Scope of Practice for Academic Nurse Educators* was first developed by the National League for Nursing's (NLN) Certification Governance Committee and published by the NLN in 2005. At that time, the leadership of the NLN and the members of the committee believed that recognition of academic nursing education as a specialty and an advanced practice nursing role was essential, and that a description of the scope and competencies of nurse educator practice and a certification exam linked to those competencies were required.

During 2010 and 2011, the NLN Certification Commission collaborated to perform an updated nurse educator practice analysis. This systematic practice analysis assessment was intended to identify any changes in the job-related responsibilities of individuals who fulfill the full scope of the nurse faculty role. The results of the 2010–2011 practice analysis resulted in slight revisions to the nurse educator certification test blueprint. The nurse educator practice analysis was again performed in 2016–2017 and 2023, each resulting in minor revisions to the nurse educator certification test blueprint.

The academic nurse educator competencies first identified pertained to the faculty member who was practicing in the full scope of the nurse educator role. But not all academic nurse educators practice in the full scope of that role. Some nurse educators focus their practice in the clinical setting. As of 2015, the role of the academic clinical nurse educator had not been described, nor had its competencies been identified. The NLN created a task group to identify the core competencies of this specific role. A practice analysis was conducted in 2016–2017 on the role of the academic clinical nurse educator, and the results were instrumental in creating the test plan for a new certification as an NLN Academic Clinical Nurse Educator. The practice analysis for the academic clinical nurse educator was repeated in 2023, resulting in minor revisions to the nurse educator certification test blueprint.

In 2021, analysis of testing data showed that nurse educators with less than two years of experience often struggled to meet the pass score on the Certified Nurse Educator examination. A task group was convened at the NLN to examine the issue and the possible need for a novice-level entry exam. The literature regarding academic novice nurse educators was reviewed, as well as the competencies. The competencies were revised to better reflect what the role of the academic novice nurse educator would be. The revisions were validated by NLN membership review and commentary. The competencies reflect the certified nurse educator competencies and have also been adjusted to the expected performance standards for a new nurse educator.

In seeking to answer if the role of the academic practical nursing and vocational nursing (PN/VN) program nurse educator should have the same competencies as the previously defined nurse educator competencies, a task force of PN/VN program nurse educators was assembled by the NLN in 2023. A literature review pertinent to the role of the academic PN/VN nurse educator was limited to 13 articles. A thematic analysis of the obtained literature identified seven themes to the role of a PN/VN nurse educator, which became competencies for this role. Task statements then were developed for each competency. A practice analysis was conducted in 2024 to verify the academic PN/VN nurse educator competencies and task statements. The results of the task group and practice analysis provided the basis for creating a competency for a test plan for another new certification specifically for the role of the NLN Academic PN/VN nurse educator.

## HISTORICAL PERSPECTIVE

The development of educational programs for the preparation of nurses parallels the evolution of nursing as a distinct profession requiring a specialized body of knowledge and skills. One of the earliest known training programs was the Deaconess Institute established in Kaiserswerth, Germany, in 1836. Deaconesses were women who promised to work for Christ by teaching or nursing. The institute became well known, and graduates of the program spread the Kaiserswerth model of care of the ill throughout the world (Donahue, 1996).

Florence Nightingale trained at the Kaiserswerth Institute in 1851. On her return to England from the Crimea in 1856, Nightingale set about achieving her two key goals: "reform of army sanitary practices and the establishment of a school for nurses" (Kalisch & Kalisch, 1995, p. 36). Today, Nightingale is credited with defining a theoretical foundation for the practice of nursing and founding the first independent, organized training program for nurses (Donahue, 1996).

In the United States, the mid-19th century saw calls for formal training of nurses by organizations such as the American Medical Association. The first training school for nurses in the United States was established in 1872 at the New England Hospital.

By 1902, there were 492 schools of nursing in the United States. Training programs expected strict discipline, long hours, and a strong focus on learning through practice. Programs began to expand from two to three years in length, and schools known for their high quality of training attracted students of increasing caliber. In 1905, Bellevue Hospital had 2,000 applicants (Kalisch & Kalisch, 1995).

During the early 20th century, most nurses were prepared in hospital-based programs. However, starting with the University of Minnesota in 1909, collegiate settings became the locus for programs of registered nursing education at the undergraduate and graduate levels. The approach to providing registered nursing education in community colleges was developed by Dr. Mildred Montag in 1949.

During this period and beyond, several important studies guided the evolution of nursing education. In 1923, the first evaluation of nursing education was published (Goldmark, 1923). Examples of other key documents include *Nurses, Patients, and Pocketbooks* in 1923; *Nursing Schools Today and Tomorrow* in 1934; *Nursing for the Future* in 1948; *Nurses for a Growing Nation* in 1957; *Toward Quality in Nursing* in 1961; *ANA Position Paper on Education for Nursing* in 1965; and *Extending the Scope of Nursing Practice* in 1971 (Kalisch & Kalisch, 1995). These documents provided important guidance to the development of nursing education in the United States and Canada.

As nursing progressed to become a profession, the science of nursing was further delineated, and the body of knowledge and skills unique to generalist and advanced practice nursing was developed and refined. Preparation of professional nurses transitioned from "training" to "education."

The first organization for nursing in the United States was officially developed in 1893. The American Society of Superintendents of Training Schools of Nurses (ASSTSN)* was formed for "the establishment and maintenance of a universal standard of training" for nursing (Fondiller, 1999).

The first formal training programs for practical nurses (PNs) were started by the Brooklyn, New York, YMCA in 1893; however, the first school was not organized until 1897.

The shortage of nurses that followed World War II prompted the expansion of PN programs, with most housed in public schools. The PN programs of today are commonly one year in length, and most PN education takes place in vocational/technical schools and community colleges (U.S. Bureau of Labor Statistics, 2025).

Although nursing education has existed for more than 160 years, academic nursing education as a specialty area of practice with a defined theoretical basis, body of knowledge, and certification has been slow to develop. Preparation of nurses as educators has occurred in graduate programs of nursing or education or through continuing education, mentoring, or experience. In order to further advance nursing education, new models of research-based nursing education must emerge. The precedent of relying on tradition and past practices must be replaced with proposed changes emanating from "evidence that substantiates the science of nursing education and provides the foundation for best educational practices" (National League for Nursing, 2005b, p. 1).

---

*The ASSTSN evolved into the National League of Nursing Education (NLNE) in 1912 and then the National League for Nursing (NLN) in 1952.

## VALUES AND BELIEFS

Academic nurse educators believe that education is a self-actualizing, creative, lifetime endeavor involving values clarification, progressive systematic inquiry, critical analysis, and judgment.

As a distinct specialty of advanced nursing practice, academic nursing education has a set of defined values and beliefs. They are evident in the NLN's *Hallmarks of Excellence*© (2020) (outlined below) and are incorporated into the standards of practice. The Hallmarks were originally published in 2004 and revised in 2020. The Hallmarks are relevant for all types of nursing programs and all types of institutions.

## NLN HALLMARKS OF EXCELLENCE©

### Hallmark # 1-1 – Engaged Students

Students are excited about learning and exhibit a spirit of inquiry as well as a commitment to lifelong learning.

### Hallmark # 1-2 – Engaged Students

Students are committed to innovation, continuous quality/performance improvement, and excellence.

### Hallmark # 1-3 – Engaged Students

Students are committed to the professional nursing role including advancement in leadership, scholarship, and mentoring.

### Hallmark # 2-1 – Diverse, Well-Prepared Faculty

The faculty complement is comprised of diverse individuals who are leaders and/or have expertise in clinical practice, education, interprofessional collaboration, and research/scholarship consistent with the parent institution's mission and vision.

### Hallmark # 2-2 – Diverse, Well-Prepared Faculty

The unique contributions of each faculty member in teaching, service, research/scholarship, and practice that facilitate achievement of the program's mission and goals are valued, rewarded, and recognized.

### Hallmark # 2-3 – Diverse, Well-Prepared Faculty

Faculty members are accountable for promoting excellence, creating civil and inclusive environments, and providing leadership in their area(s) of expertise.

## Hallmark # 2-4 – Diverse, Well-Prepared Faculty

Faculty members model a commitment to lifelong learning, involvement in professional and community organizations, and scholarly activities.

## Hallmark # 2-5 – Diverse, Well-Prepared Faculty

All faculty members have structured preparation for the faculty role, including competence in teaching, scholarship, and service.

## Hallmark # 3-1 – A Culture of Continuous Quality Improvement

The program engages in a variety of activities that promote quality and excellence, including accreditation by national nursing accreditation bodies.

## Hallmark # 3-2 – A Culture of Continuous Quality Improvement

Program design, implementation, and evaluation are continuously reviewed and revised to achieve and maintain excellence.

## Hallmark # 4-1 – Innovative, Evidence-Based Curriculum

The curriculum is designed to help students achieve stated program outcomes, reflects current societal and health care trends and issues, and is responsive to change and evolving societal needs. The curriculum also embeds evidence-based information, reflects research findings and innovative practices, attends to the evolving role of the nurse in a variety of settings, is flexible and innovative, and incorporates local, national, and global perspectives.

## Hallmark # 4-2 – Innovative, Evidence-Based Curriculum

The curriculum provides learning activities that enhance students' abilities to think critically, reflect thoughtfully, and provide culturally sensitive, evidence-based nursing care to diverse populations.

## Hallmark # 4-3 – Innovative, Evidence-Based Curriculum

The curriculum emphasizes students' values development, identity formation, caring for self, commitment to lifelong learning, critical thinking, ethical and evidence-based practice, and creativity.

## Hallmark # 4-4 – Innovative, Evidence-Based Curriculum

The curriculum provides learning experiences that prepare graduates to assume roles that are essential to quality nursing practice, including but not limited to roles of care provider, advocate for those in need, teacher, communicator, change agent, care coordinator, member of intra- and interprofessional teams, user of information technology, collaborator, decision-maker, leader, and evolving scholar.

## Hallmark # 4-5 – Innovative, Evidence-Based Curriculum

The curriculum provides learning experiences that support evidence-based practice, interprofessional approaches to care, student achievement of clinical competence, and, as appropriate, competence in a specialty role.

## Hallmark # 5-1 – Innovative, Evidence-Based Approaches to Facilitate and Evaluate Learning

Strategies used to facilitate and evaluate learning by a diverse student population are innovative and varied.

## Hallmark # 5-2 – Innovative, Evidence-Based Approaches to Facilitate and Evaluate Learning

Faculty members engage in collegial dialogue and interact with students and colleagues in nursing and other professions to promote and develop strategies to facilitate and evaluate learning.

## Hallmark # 5-3 – Innovative, Evidence-Based Approaches to Facilitate and Evaluate Learning

Strategies to facilitate and evaluate learning used by faculty members are evidence based.

## Hallmark # 6-1 – Resources to Support Program Goal Attainment

Partnerships in which the program is engaged promote excellence in nursing education, enhance the profession, benefit the community, enhance learning opportunities, and facilitate/support research/scholarship initiatives.

## Hallmark # 6-2 – Resources to Support Program Goal Attainment

Technology is used effectively to facilitate, support, and evaluate student learning, faculty development, research/scholarship, and support services.

## Hallmark # 6-3 – Resources to Support Program Goal Attainment

Student support services are culturally sensitive and empower students during the recruitment, retention, progression, graduation, and career planning processes.

## Hallmark # 6-4 – Resources to Support Program Goal Attainment

Financial resources are available to support initiatives that enhance faculty competence, student success, innovation, and scholarly endeavors.

## Hallmark # 7-1 – Commitment to Pedagogical Scholarship

Faculty members and students contribute to the development of the science of nursing education through the critique, use, dissemination, and/or conduct of various forms of scholarly endeavors.

## Hallmark # 7-2 – Commitment to Pedagogical Scholarship

Faculty members and students explore the influence of student learning experiences on the health of the individuals and populations they serve in various health care settings.

## Hallmark # 8-1 – Effective Institutional and Professional Leadership

Faculty members, administrators, and students provide the leadership needed to ensure that the culture of the school promotes excellence and a healthy work environment characterized by collegial dialogue, innovation, change, creativity, values development, and ethical behavior.

## Hallmark # 8-2 – Effective Institutional and Professional Leadership

Faculty members, administrators, students, and alumni are respected as leaders in the parent institution, as well as in local, state, regional, national, and/or international communities.

## Hallmark # 8-3 – Effective Institutional and Professional Leadership

Faculty members, administrators, students, and alumni are prepared for and assume leadership roles that advance quality nursing care; promote positive change, innovation, and excellence; and enhance the impact of the nursing profession.

# THEORETICAL FOUNDATIONS

*Nursing: Scope and Standards of Practice, Third Edition* (American Nurses Association [ANA], 2015), builds on previous work and provides the following contemporary definition of nursing: "Nursing is the protection, promotion, and optimization of health and abilities, prevention of illness and injury, facilitation of healing, alleviation of suffering through the diagnosis and treatment of human response, and advocacy in the care of individuals, families, groups, communities, and populations" (p. 7).

As a specialty area of advanced nursing practice, academic nursing education has a theoretical foundation that includes models and theories from nursing science, "educational psychology, instructional technology, instructional design, tests and measurement, and evaluation theory" (Caputi & Engelmann, 2004, p. 3).

Several models and theories have been used to develop the scope and standards of practice in the academic nurse educator role that are relevant to faculty teaching in all types of nursing programs: PN/VN, associate degree, diploma, baccalaureate, master's degree, and doctorate. Examples of models and theories from education with relevance for nursing education include Boyer's scholarship of engagement (Boyer, 1990), Kolb's learning cycle (Kolb, 1984), Bloom's taxonomy of learning objectives (Krathwohl et al., 1964), learning theories such as Knowles's adult learning theory (Knowles et al., 1998), community-academic partnerships (Tagliareni & Marckx, 1997), and service learning (Community Campus Partnerships for Health, n.d.).

Boyer (1990) described a perspective of the scholarly role of faculty that went beyond the traditional interpretation of research as the "only way to increase the knowledge of the discipline and as the only means for incentive and compensation of the academic professional" (Kirkpatrick & Valley, 2004). He outlined four types of scholarship in which faculty engage: discovery (disciplined investigative efforts leading to new knowledge), integration (synthesis, making connections across disciplines), application (using knowledge in implementing a practice role or in service to the larger community), and teaching (transmitting, transforming, and extending knowledge). The extent to which a particular academic nurse educator engages in each type of scholarship will vary in accord with factors such as her/his professional goals and the type of program in which she/he teaches.

## EXPLORATION OF ACADEMIC NURSE EDUCATOR ROLES: FROM EVIDENCE-BASED FOUNDATIONS TO CERTIFICATIONS

The exploration of the different nurse educator roles follows a defined process. The first step is the establishment of a task group with the primary defined goal of reviewing literature to search for what is known about the role. The findings of the literature are analyzed and synthesized into an overall description of the role. The findings also lend themselves to identifying themes within the role. The task group reviews and discusses the themes with the next goal of using the themes to establish defined competencies for that role.

Once the themes of the role have been identified, the task group's activities then focus on identifying task statements, again derived from the relevant literature findings for the role. Each competency will be supported by and further described by a set of related task statements. These task statements include day-to-day activities in teaching and being a faculty member. Attention also is given to professional development and other activities that nurse educators regularly perform.

When the competencies and task statements are delineated sufficiently to be approved by the task group, a survey is constructed to verify the newly identified role competencies and task statements from those currently engaged in the role. The survey participants are asked to rate (in different ways) the regularity of the task and importance of the task to the role. These data lead to validation of the work of the task group that the role has been accurately defined. The analysis of the data also leads to revisions of the competencies and task statements.

The next step is the creation of a survey known as a practice analysis. The step of completing the practice analysis involves a committee of subject matter experts, along with a consulting psychometrician. The purpose of the practice analysis is to identify the frequency and importance of each competency and task statement by nurse educators currently engaged in the role. The data collected are analyzed once again and can further validate or lead to revisions of the competencies and task statements. Ultimately, the final result of the practice analysis is to have a statistically valid certification test blueprint based on the perceived significance of the tasks of the role.

Experts in the role then create relevant test items that correlate to the test blueprint. All test items are edited by additional role experts. Various forms of the exam will be created from the developed and edited test bank of items. All test items are pilot tested by a group of persons engaged in the identified nurse educator role. The data from the pilot test are reviewed by item analysis to assure each individual item meets certain psychometric quality indicators. Any test items not meeting preset quality analysis indicators will be revised or deleted.

After the pilot period closes, the process moves to the test development committee identifying a cut score or *passing score*. Using psychometric procedures, a passing score for each form of the exam is set. At times, there may be two or more forms of the exam, each having the same passing score or possibly slightly different passing scores. If exam forms have different passing scores, it is the result of psychometric determination that one form of the exam may be slightly more difficult than another form. A more difficult form of the exam may have a slightly lower passing score.

The final step in the certification exam development involves more review by content experts and consensus that the examination forms are sound, psychometrically developed, valid, and reliable. The exams are released as the tool for determining who becomes certified and who is not successful.

Beginning with the practice analysis step, all the certification exams move through this same process every five years. Repeating the same process for practice verification ensures that practice changes within the nurse educator role are identified and certification testing of the role remains current.

# 2

# The Academic Nurse Educator Practicing in the Full Scope of the Role

## DEFINITION

### Academic Nurse Educator in the Full Scope of the Role

Academic nursing education is the process of facilitating learning through curriculum design, teaching, evaluation, advisement, and other activities undertaken by faculty in schools of nursing. Academic nursing education is a specialty area and an advanced practice role within professional nursing.

Academic nurse educators engage in many roles and functions, each of which reflects the core competencies of nursing faculty. The extent to which a specific nurse educator implements these competencies varies according to many factors, including the mission of the nurse educator's institution, the nurse educator's academic rank and academic preparation, and the type of program in which the nurse educator teaches. The academic nurse educator engaged in all the core competencies is practicing in the full scope of the role.

## SCOPE OF PRACTICE

"The scope of practice statement describes the 'who, what, where, when, why, and how' of nursing practice" (American Nurses Association [ANA], 2017, p. 14). The term "academic nurse educator" refers to an individual who fulfills a faculty role in an academic setting. In nursing, this role is implemented in practical nursing and vocational nursing (PN/VN), registered nursing (RN), and graduate programs.

Whereas individuals with appointments to a nursing faculty may hold advanced preparation in disciplines supportive to nursing (e.g., nutrition and pharmacology), the scope of practice described here relates to individuals with advanced preparation in nursing who teach nursing courses. "Competence as an educator can be established, recognized, and expanded through master's and/or doctoral education, post-master's certificate programs, continuing professional development, mentoring activities, and professional certification as a faculty member" (National League for Nursing [NLN], 2002, p. 4).

Nursing education takes place in diverse settings that include, but are not limited to, technical schools, hospitals, two- and four-year colleges, and universities. The implementation of the academic faculty role may occur in traditional classroom-based environments or in nontraditional environments.

Academic nurse educators engage in multiple roles and functions, each of which reflects the core competencies of nursing faculty. The NLN (2005a) identified nurse educator competencies as the following: (1) facilitate learning, (2) facilitate learner development and socialization, (3) use assessment and evaluation strategies, (4) participate in curriculum design and evaluation of program outcomes, (5) function as a change agent and leader, (6) pursue continuous quality improvement in the nurse educator role, (7) engage in scholarship, and (8) function within the educational environment. The extent to which a specific nurse educator implements these competencies varies according to many factors, including the mission of her/his institution, rank, academic preparation, and the type of program in which she/he is teaching.

The development of a master nurse educator evolves over time. To that end, it is recognized that a nurse educator can function at a competent level early in her/his career, but mastery occurs with guidance, ongoing professional development, and practice.

## STANDARDS OF PRACTICE

Standards of practice are considered authoritative duties that nurses are expected to perform competently (American Nurses Association [ANA], 2017). The ANA further identified two categories of standards: "a) Standards of Practice that describe a competent level of nursing practice as demonstrated by the nursing process, and b) Standards of Professional Performance that describe a competent level of behavior in the professional role" (ANA, 2017, p. 4).

An academic nurse educator is a professional role within nursing. The following core competencies identify the diverse duties that have become the standards of professional role performance for academic nurse educators practicing in the full scope of the role.

## CORE COMPETENCIES OF ACADEMIC NURSE EDUCATORS WITH TASK STATEMENTS

### Competency 1: Facilitate Learning

- Implement a variety of active teaching and learning strategies appropriate to content concepts, setting, learner attribute and needs, learner outcomes, and method of delivery.
- Use teaching and learning strategies based on educational theories and evidence-based practices related to education.
- Modify teaching strategies and learning experiences based on consideration of learners' diversity, social determinants of learning, and past clinical, education, and life experiences.
- Use technologies to support the teaching–learning process.
- Communicate effectively to convey ideas in a variety of contexts.
- Model reflective thinking practices.
- Create opportunities for learners to develop clinical judgment.

- Ensure a positive and safe learning environment.
- Model attributes that facilitate learning.
- Develop and maintain effective working relationships with health care and education partners.
- Apply concepts of evidence-based practice in nursing to guide teaching.

## Competency 2: Facilitate Learner Development and Socialization

- Identify learner attributes and needs based on consideration of learners' diversity, social determinants of learning, and past clinical, educational, and life experiences.
- Facilitate access to various resources to support diverse learners.
- Assist learners to identify and develop a plan to meet professional goals.
- Facilitate learners' self-reflection, goal setting, and socialization to the role of the nurse.
- Engage learners in thoughtful and constructive self and peer evaluation.
- Promote professional development of learners.

## Competency 3: Use Assessment and Evaluation Strategies

- Design and apply formative and summative evaluation strategies.
- Implement evidence-based strategies in cognitive, psychomotor, and affective learning domains.
- Evaluate available methods for learner assessment and evaluation.
- Create assessment methods that evaluate outcomes.
- Implement evaluation methods that are congruent with learner and learning outcomes.
- Analyze assessment and evaluation data.
- Apply assessment and evaluation data to enhance the teaching–learning process.
- Inform learners about assessment and evaluation criteria.
- Provide timely, constructive, and thoughtful feedback to learners.

## Competency 4: Participate in Curriculum Design and Evaluation of Program Outcomes

- Provide input for the development of nursing program standards and policies regarding admission, progression, retention, and graduation.
- Demonstrate knowledge of curriculum development, including developing program outcomes and/or competency statements, writing content objectives and course outcomes, selecting learning activities and clinical experiences consistent with course outcomes, and designing evaluation strategies consistent with course and program outcomes.

- Design curriculum to reflect institutional philosophy and mission; current nursing and health care trends; community, clinical partners, and societal needs; nursing principles, standards, theory, research, and innovation; use of technology; and mode of educational delivery.
- Lead the development of curriculum design.
- Lead the development of course design.
- Design program evaluation that promotes continuous quality improvement.
- Implement the program evaluation plan.
- Analyze results of program evaluation.
- Revise the curriculum based on evaluation of program outcomes, learner needs, societal and health care trends, and stakeholder feedback.
- Implement curricular revisions using change theories and evidence-based strategies.
- Evaluate the program evaluation plan.

## Competency 5: Function as a Change Agent and Leader

- Evaluate organizational effectiveness to determine the needed change.
- Adapt to changes created by external factors.
- Create a culture of change within the nursing program and institution.
- Design, implement, and evaluate strategies for change.
- Model principles of diversity, equity, and inclusivity when advocating for change.
- Serve as a leader to promote nursing and nursing education.
- Facilitate interprofessional education and collaboration to impact health and educational outcomes.
- Manage conflict effectively.

## Competency 6: Pursue Continuous Quality Improvement in the Nurse Educator Role

- Participate actively in professional nursing and educational organizations.
- Demonstrate a commitment to lifelong learning.
- Use feedback gained from self, peer, student, and administrative evaluation to improve role effectiveness.
- Stay current with legal standards and ethical codes relevant to nursing and educational settings.
- Remain informed with health care policy relevant to nursing and educational settings.
- Seek mentors for professional development in the academic nurse educator role.
- Engage in self-reflection and self-care to improve teaching practices.

## Competency 7: Engage in Scholarship

- Foster a culture of scholarly inquiry.
- Demonstrate qualities of a scholar.
- Disseminate the outcomes of scholarly activities.

## Competency 8: Function Within the Educational Environment

- Analyze the impact of social, technological, economic, political, and institutional factors on nursing and nursing education.
- Apply knowledge of historical and current trends and issues to decision-making in nursing and nursing education.
- Integrate the values of civility, collegiality, professionalism, and caring to build an organizational climate that fosters the development of learners and colleagues.
- Demonstrate the support of diversity, equity, and inclusion initiatives to align with the organization's mission and vision.
- Incorporate the mission and goals of the nursing program and the parent institution when managing issues.
- Manage the teaching, scholarship, and service demands congruent with the requirements of the institutional setting.
- Serve as a leader in governance and activities within the nursing program and/or the parent institution.
- Use social media in a manner consistent with professional and institutional guidelines.
- Provide input into the budgetary processes of the program and parent institution.
- Maintain professional role boundaries as an educator.

# 3

# The Academic Nurse Educator Practicing Within the Clinical Educator Role

## DEFINITION

### Academic Clinical Nurse Educator

According to the *NLN Certified Academic Clinical Nurse Educator (CNE®cl) 2024 Candidate Handbook*, "[T]he academic clinical nurse educator facilitates the learning of nursing students throughout clinical components of an academic nursing program. This educator is guided in this role by faculty of the nursing program and is accountable to that nursing program for providing fair evaluations of learners' performance in meeting expected learning outcomes. The academic clinical nurse educator may have a variety of titles depending upon the classification used by the specific nursing education program (e.g., clinical faculty, part-time faculty, adjunct faculty, clinical instructor, preceptor)" (National League for Nursing [NLN], 2024, p. 2).

## SCOPE OF PRACTICE

The academic clinical nurse educator has experience within professional nursing practice and academic nursing education practice. Within professional nursing practice, the academic clinical nurse educator has gained competence in nursing practice and can share this competence with students in the clinical components of academic nursing education.

The academic clinical nurse educator also "has experience as an educator in an academic setting and responsibility for facilitating student learning (in the laboratory and/or clinical setting). This experience may be with learners enrolled in pre- or post-licensure nursing programs" (NLN, 2024, p. 2).

The academic clinical nurse educator's role varies from other clinical educator roles, such as the traditional hospital-based clinical nurse educator who provides employee orientation and staff development. The academic clinical nurse educator "reports to the school/department of nursing about learner performance in clinical settings, submits evaluations about the performance of learners receiving academic credit for the clinical learning experience, and supervises the learner in the setting" (NLN, 2024, p. 3). This role is accountable for selecting appropriate clinical learning experiences and providing support for the learner to meet the expected clinical outcomes.

# STANDARDS OF PRACTICE

The academic clinical nurse educator is a professional role within nursing. The following core competencies reflect the standards of professional role performance for the academic clinical nurse educator.

# CORE COMPETENCIES OF ACADEMIC CLINICAL NURSE EDUCATORS WITH TASK STATEMENTS

## Competency 1: Function Within the Education and Health Care Environments

A. **Function in the Clinical Educator Role**

- Bridge the gap between theory and practice by helping learners apply classroom learning to the clinical setting.
- Foster the professional growth of learners.
- Use technologies to enhance clinical teaching and learning.
- Value the contributions of others in the achievement of learner outcomes.
- Act as a role model of professional nursing within the clinical learning environment.
- Demonstrate inclusive excellence.

B. **Operationalize the Curriculum**

- Assess the congruence of the clinical agency to the curriculum, core goals, and learner needs.
- Plan meaningful and relevant clinical learning assignments and activities.
- Identify learners' goals and outcomes.
- Prepare learners for clinical experiences.
- Structure learner experiences within the learning environment to promote optimal learning.
- Implement clinical learning activities to help learners develop interprofessional collaboration and teamwork skills.
- Provide opportunities for learners to develop problem-solving and clinical reasoning skills related to learning outcomes.
- Implement assigned models for clinical teaching.
- Engage in theory-based instruction.
- Provide input to the nursing program for course development and review.

C. **Abide by Legal Requirements, Ethical Guidelines, Agency Policies, and Guiding Framework**

- Apply ethical and legal principles to create a safe clinical learning environment.
- Assess learner abilities and needs prior to clinical learning experiences.

- Facilitate learning activities that support the mission, goals, and values of the academic institution and the clinical agency.
- Inform others of program and clinical agency policies, procedures, and practices.
- Adhere to program and clinical agency policies, procedures, and practices when implementing clinical experiences.
- Promote learner compliance with regulations and standards of practice.
- Demonstrate ethical behaviors.

## Competency 2: Facilitate Learning in the Health Care Environment

- Implement a variety of clinical teaching strategies congruent with learner needs, desired learner outcomes, content, and context.
- Ground teaching strategies in educational theory and evidence-based teaching practices.
- Use technology skillfully to support the teaching–learning process.
- Create opportunities for learners to develop critical thinking and clinical reasoning skills.
- Promote a culture of safety and quality in the health care environment.
- Create a positive and caring learning environment.
- Develop collegial working relationships with learners, faculty colleagues, and clinical agency personnel.
- Demonstrate enthusiasm for teaching, learning, and nursing to help inspire and motivate learners.

## Competency 3: Demonstrate Effective Interpersonal Communication and Collaborative Interprofessional Relationships

- Value collaboration and coordination of care.
- Foster a shared learning community, and cooperate with other members of the health care team.
- Support an environment of frequent, respectful, civil, and open communication with all members of the health care team.
- Act as a role model showing respect for all members of the health care team, professional colleagues, clients, family members, as well as learners.
- Use clear and effective communication in all interactions.
- Listen to learner concerns, needs, or questions in a nonthreatening way.
- Display a calm, empathetic, and supportive demeanor in all communications.
- Manage emotions effectively when communicating in challenging situations.

- Effectively manage conflict.
- Maintain an approachable, nonjudgmental, and readily accessible demeanor.
- Recognize limitations in self and learners to provide opportunities for development.
- Demonstrate effective communication in clinical learning environments with diverse colleagues, clients, cultures, health care professionals, and learners.
- Communicate performance expectations to learners and agency staff.

## Competency 4: Apply Clinical Expertise in the Health Care Environment

- Maintain current professional competence relevant to the specialty area, practice setting, and clinical learning environment.
- Translate theory into clinical practice by applying experiential knowledge and clinical reasoning, and using a client-centered approach to clinical instruction.
- Use best evidence to address client-related problems.
- Demonstrate effective leadership within the clinical learning environment.
- Demonstrate sound clinical reasoning.
- Expand knowledge and skills by integrating best practices.
- Balance client care needs and student learning needs within a culture of safety.
- Demonstrate competence with a range of technologies available in the clinical learning environment.

## Competency 5: Facilitate Learner Development and Socialization

- Mentor learners in the development of professional nursing behaviors, standards, and codes of ethics.
- Promote a learning climate of respect for all.
- Promote professional integrity and accountability.
- Maintain professional boundaries.
- Encourage ongoing learner professional development via formal and informal venues.
- Assist learners in effective use of self-assessment and professional goal setting for ongoing self-improvement.
- Create learning environments that are focused on socialization to the role of the nurse.
- Assist learners to develop the ability to engage in constructive peer feedback.
- Inspire creativity and confidence.
- Encourage various techniques for learners to develop the ability to engage in constructive peer feedback.
- Inspire creativity and confidence.

- Encourage various techniques for learners to manage stress.
- Act as a role model for self-reflection, self-care, and coping skills.
- Empower learners to be successful in meeting professional and educational goals.
- Engage learners in applying best practices and quality improvement processes.

## Competency 6: Implement Effective Clinical and Assessment Evaluation Strategies

- Use a variety of strategies to determine achievement of learning outcomes.
- Implement both formative and summative evaluation that is appropriate to the learner and learner outcomes.
- Engage in timely communication with course faculty regarding learner clinical performance.
- Maintain integrity in the assessment and evaluation of learners.
- Provide timely, objective, constructive, and fair feedback to learners.
- Use learner data to enhance the teaching–learning process in the clinical learning environment.
- Demonstrate skill in the use of best practices in the assessment and evaluation of clinical performance.
- Assess and evaluate learner achievement of clinical performance expectations.
- Use performance standards to determine learner strengths and weaknesses in the clinical learning environment.
- Document learner clinical performance, feedback, and progression.
- Evaluate the quality of the clinical learning experiences and environment.

# 4

# The Academic Nurse Educator Practicing Within the Novice Role

## DEFINITION

### Academic Novice Nurse Educator

In practice, the role of the academic novice nurse educator is often not synchronized with the expectations of academic nurse educators functioning within the full scope of the role. While most of the task statements from the academic nurse educator role are applicable, the academic novice nurse educator may not perform the task at the same level but more at a novice, or new nurse, educator level. The novice level is defined as new faculty with less than three years of experience as an academic nurse educator.

## SCOPE OF PRACTICE

The academic novice nurse educator's role encompasses the same broad expectations of an academic nurse educator functioning in the full scope of the role. However, the novice role reflects a new nurse educator who is not yet expected to perform at the same level as a more experienced academic nurse educator.

## STANDARDS OF PRACTICE

The academic novice nurse educator is a professional role within nursing. The following core competencies reflect the standards of professional role performance for the academic novice nurse educator.

## CORE COMPETENCIES OF ACADEMIC NOVICE NURSE EDUCATORS WITH TASK STATEMENTS

### Competency 1: Facilitate Learning

- Implement a variety of active teaching and learning strategies appropriate to content/concepts, setting, learner attribute and needs, learner outcomes, and method of delivery.

- Use teaching and learning strategies based on educational theories and evidence-based practices related to education.
- Engage in self-reflection and continued learning to improve teaching practices that facilitate learning.
- Use technologies skillfully to support the teaching–learning process.
- Use oral, written, and electronic communication that reflects an awareness of self and others, along with an ability to convey ideas in a variety of contexts.
- Engage in critical and reflective thinking, considering multiple perspectives.
- Provide opportunities for learners to develop critical thinking and clinical judgment skills.
- Show enthusiasm for teaching, learning, and nursing that inspires and motivates learners.
- Use personal attributes (e.g., caring, confidence, patience, integrity, flexibility) that facilitate learning.
- Participate positively in collegial working relationships with learners, faculty colleagues, and the interprofessional health care team to promote learning.
- Maintain the professional practice knowledge base needed to assist learners to prepare for contemporary nursing practice.
- Serve as a role model of professional nursing.
- Create a physically, psychologically, emotionally safe learning environment.
- Establish professional boundaries.

## Competency 2: Facilitate Learner Development and Socialization

- Recognize individual learning and professional socialization needs of diverse learner populations.
- Identify resources available for diverse learners that assist in meeting individual learning needs.
- Describe the advisement and counseling processes to support learners in the achievement of professional goals.
- Guide learner self-reflection and personal goal setting.
- Foster the cognitive, psychomotor, and affective development of learners.
- Recognize the influence of teaching strategies and communication on learner outcomes.
- Encourage learners to engage in thoughtful and constructive self-evaluation.
- Discuss the importance of involvement in professional organizations and a commitment to lifelong learning in pursuit of professional role development.
- Communicate the value of interprofessional practice and collaboration among members of the health care team.
- Recognize the influences that social determinants of education have on teaching and learning.

## Competency 3: Use Assessment and Evaluation Strategies

- Use extant literature to develop evidence-based assessment and evaluation practices.
- Employ a variety of strategies to assess and evaluate learning in cognitive, psychomotor, and affective domains.
- Implement formative and summative evidence-based assessment and evaluation strategies.
- Enhance the teaching–learning process based upon data.
- Provide timely, constructive, and thoughtful feedback to learners.

## Competency 4: Participate in Curriculum Design and Evaluation of Program Outcomes

- Identify that the curriculum reflects the institutional philosophy and mission; current nursing and health care trends; and community/social needs that prepare graduates for practice in a complex, dynamic, diverse health care environment.
- Recognize the influences of accreditation and regulatory standards on curriculum development.
- Demonstrate knowledge of curriculum development, including identification of program outcomes, development of competency statements, writing learning outcomes, and selecting learning activities and evaluation strategies.
- Relate curriculum design and implementation decisions to sound educational principles, theory, and research.
- Contribute to curriculum revision based on assessment of program outcomes, learner needs, and societal and health care trends.
- Use appropriate change theories and strategies when implementing curricular revisions.
- Assist in maintaining community and clinical partnerships that support educational goals.
- Collaborate with external constituencies regarding curriculum and evaluation of program outcomes.
- Provide program assessment and evaluation data to promote continuous quality improvement of all aspects of the program.

## Competency 5: Function as a Change Agent and Leader

- Demonstrate cultural humility when advocating for change.
- Develop an inclusive, innovative, and creative perspective of the nurse educator role.
- Recognize interprofessional efforts to address health care, health policy, and educational needs locally, regionally, nationally, and internationally.

- Describe the influence of organization effectiveness in nursing education.
- Identify strategies for organizational change.
- Explain the leadership structure in the nursing program and parent institution.
- Incorporate innovative practices in educational environments.
- Develop leadership behaviors for shaping and implementing change.

## Competency 6: Pursue Continuous Quality Improvement in the Nurse Educator Role

- Demonstrate a commitment to lifelong learning.
- Recognize that career enhancement needs and activities change as experience is gained in the role.
- Engage in professional development opportunities that increase one's effectiveness in the role.
- Describe the teaching, scholarship, and service demands inherent in the role of educator and member of the academic institution.
- Use feedback gained from self, peer, learner, and/or administrative evaluation to improve role effectiveness.
- Use knowledge of legal and ethical issues relevant to higher education and nursing education.
- Seek mentors to enhance development in the role.

## Competency 7: Engage in Scholarship

- Draw on extant literature to design evidence-based teaching practices.
- Exhibit a spirit of inquiry about teaching and learning, learner development, evaluation methods, and other aspects of the role.
- Design and implement scholarly activities in an established area of expertise.
- Disseminate nursing and teaching knowledge to a variety of audiences through multiple means.
- Demonstrate attributes of a scholar of integrity, courage, perseverance, vitality, and creativity.

## Competency 8: Function Within the Educational Environment

- Identify history, current trends, issues, roles, and boundaries in higher education.
- Identify how social, technological, economic, political, and institutional forces impact higher education in general and nursing education specifically.
- Engage in cross-mentorship (mentor–mentee), collaborations, and partnerships.
- Participate in academic, professional, and community service.

- Develop professional goals that align with the nursing program and the parent institution.
- Integrate the values of civility, collegiality, professionalism, and caring to build an organizational climate that fosters the development of learners and nurse educators.
- Support the goals and mission of the nursing program and the parent institution when managing conflict.
- Implement policies and procedures related to learners, faculty, and the educational environment.
- Discuss the various levels of governance, including shared governance, within the nursing program and the parent institution.
- Use social media in a manner consistent with professional and institutional guidelines.
- Describe the role of faculty input into the budgetary processes of the program and parent institution.
- Maintain professional role boundaries as an educator.

# 5

# The Academic Nurse Educator Practicing Within the Practical/ Vocational Program Role

## DEFINITION

### Academic Nurse Educator Practicing Within the PN/VN Nurse Educator Role

The academic practical nursing and vocational nursing (PN/VN) nurse educator delivers basic nursing education to practical and vocational learners. The basic nursing education includes content and skills delivery, as well as assessment and evaluation of learner performance.

## SCOPE OF PRACTICE

The academic PN/VN nurse educator has experience within professional nursing practice and engagement in nursing education practice. Within professional nursing practice, the academic PN/VN nurse educator has gained competence in nursing practice and can share this competence with students in the clinical components of academic nursing education.

The academic PN/VN nurse educator demonstrates responsibility for facilitating student learning in the classroom, laboratory, and clinical settings. The educator understands and adheres to regulatory guidelines and state practice acts.

The academic PN/VN nurse educator's role varies from other nurse educator roles, as evidenced in the defined competencies and task statements. This role is accountable for delivering classroom content, selecting clinical learning experiences, and providing support for the learner to meet the expected clinical outcomes.

## STANDARDS OF PRACTICE

The academic nurse educator practicing within the PN/VN nurse educator role is a professional role within nursing. The following core competencies reflect the standards of professional role performance for the academic nurse educator practicing within the PN/VN program role.

# CORE COMPETENCIES OF THE ACADEMIC PRACTICAL/VOCATIONAL PROGRAM NURSE EDUCATORS WITH TASK STATEMENTS

## Competency 1: Facilitates Learning

- Effectively promote learning of concepts and evidence-based content in a fast-paced delivery pathway.
- Demonstrate a firm knowledge base of theory and evidence-based teaching strategies.
- Implement learner-centered teaching strategies.
- Integrate effective use of the curriculum components.
- Develop and maintain professionalism with learning partnership.
- Provide quality and safe clinical experiences that correlate with course and program outcomes.
- Use effective and successful coaching techniques with learners.
- Demonstrate an in-depth knowledge of the role of the practical/vocational nurse.
- Is knowledgeable about legal and ethical issues related to the practice of practical/vocational nurses.
- Effectively use technology to enhance the teaching/learning process.
- Is knowledgeable on multiple levels about regulatory issues that impact nursing.
- Effectively address the learning needs of diverse learner populations.
- Instruct in constructs of self-awareness and self-reflection.

## Competency 2: Provides Assessment and Evaluation of Learners

- Use a variety of formative and summative assessment and evaluation tools.
- Demonstrate the use of reliability and validity concepts when measuring learner achievement.
- Demonstrate proficiency in the leveling of assessment materials.
- Show ability in and use of various methodologies of assessment.
- Provide effective and timely feedback in oral and written forms.
- Use resources of peer review and colleague collaboration when indicated.
- Effectively use available assessment technologies.
- Offer feedback related to revision of assessment and evaluation tools.
- Demonstrate use of testing blueprints, testing development, testing procedures, and item analysis data.

## Competency 3: Participates in Program Evaluation and Revision

- Demonstrate understanding of a systematic plan of evaluation and related processes.

- Effectively design course and program outcomes that align with organizational goals.
- Participate in continuous evaluation and quality improvement initiatives.
- Is knowledgeable about program accreditation standards and the impact on program evaluation and revision.
- Participate in curriculum development and revision activities.

## Competency 4: Collaborates with Partners in the Learning Environment

- Demonstrate professional communication, interpersonal relationships, and teamwork.
- Effectively use communication with clinical personnel and internal and external stakeholders.
- Validate course and program outcomes with clinical partner input.
- Employ outcomes of data from learner performance evaluations and feedback by stakeholders.
- Demonstrate role-modeling skills with learners and staff in clinical settings.
- Provide an orientation to clinical site facilities with learners.
- Facilitate learner acculturation into various clinical settings.
- Support learner experiences with clinical staff and care assignments.
- Ensure that multidisciplinary contributions are integrated into didactic and clinical content.
- Share and adhere to regulatory standards.

## Competency 5: Fosters a Positive Learning Environment

- Create a caring and safe environment for learning.
- Be approachable, caring, and respectful to learners and staff of the clinical setting.
- Role model as a nurse educator.
- Ensure open and safe communication.
- Demonstrate connection, inclusivity, and ethical behaviors in the learning environment.
- Apply knowledge about and employ adult learning principles.
- Monitor group dynamics, and create a caring and sharing environment for learners.
- Reinforce clinical judgment through reflection and discussion.
- Role model behaviors of self-awareness and self-reflection.
- Monitor and maintain confidentiality in all settings.
- Identify legal issues in nursing education (i.e., use of social media).
- Foster a culture of civility in all interactions.

## Competency 6: Supports the Program and Organization

- Advocate for nursing and nursing education.
- Demonstrate willingness to serve on committees (program, organizational, community).
- Help to create and adhere to program policies and procedures.
- Identify current trends in nursing and nursing education.
- Ensure due process within the program.
- Participate in establishing and supporting a just culture within the program.
- Perform program activities as assigned (i.e., advising, mentoring).
- Provide support of colleagues for mentoring and socialization into the program and organizational culture.
- Contribute and adhere to program policies and procedures.

## Competency 7: Engages in Professional Development

- Current in the use of professional standards, evidence-based resources, and clinical practice.
- Engage and actively participate in professional organization memberships.
- Pursue micro-credentialing activities or professional certifications.
- Value the importance of continuous professional growth.
- Seek continuous educational opportunities to enhance personal growth and professional development.
- Role model self-care practices.

# 6

# Literature Focused on Academic Nurse Educator Roles

Since the National League for Nursing (NLN) identified the core competencies of the academic nurse educator in 2005, the competencies have been integrated within nursing education in various ways. The competencies have been the basis for promoting education within the faculty role through their integration into graduate nursing education curricula and nursing faculty continuing education offerings (Christensen & Halstead, 2019). The NLN academic nurse educator competencies also have been integrated into the position descriptions of nurse educators and their performance evaluations (Christensen & Halstead, 2019). Use of the core competencies as the framework for nurse educator orientation programs was suggested by Danna et al. (2010).

Despite the use of the NLN academic nurse educator competencies, little research had been conducted related to this role or the competencies as of 2015 (Christensen, 2015); this gap remains today. Such research can be identified as qualitative studies, studies focusing on Certified Nurse Educator (CNE®) exam outcomes, descriptive studies of the perceived competence of nurse educators, and quasi-experimental studies (Frenn & Dreifuerst, 2019).

The NLN core competencies of the academic clinical nurse educator have only recently been identified. As a result, very little can be found in the literature focused on the academic clinical nurse educator competencies, and no research related to these competencies can be identified.

The NLN's research agenda promotes the role of nurse scientists and calls for nurse scholars to "build the science of nursing education through the generation and translation of innovative teaching and learning strategies" (NLN, n.d.). Future research related to the academic nurse educator competencies could focus on answering questions such as the following: Does faculty competency attainment impact faculty performance and student outcomes, do self-ratings of CNEs correlate significantly with interrater-evaluated ratings as to attainment of core competencies, and what are the priority competencies for nurse educators teaching in a variety of different program types (Frenn & Dreifuerst, 2019)? Academic clinical nurse educator competency research could initially focus on descriptive studies of those who attain certification and on qualitative studies.

A limited number of research and nonresearch publications have been included in the NLN's research journal *Nursing Education Perspectives* (NEP). A summary of NEP publications is included in Appendix A. NEP publications focused on the academic nurse educator role and certification include article abstracts, the "President's Message," "NEP Quick Reads," and "Headlines from the NLN."

# 7

# The Future for Academic Nurse Educator Roles: Final Thoughts

Nursing education is a dynamic field that is experiencing the challenges of a nursing faculty shortage, increasingly sophisticated technologies, and the stimulation of a diverse student population. Clinical competence and educational expertise are required to continue the advancement of the specialty. The influence of evidence-based practice and new research in nursing education, successful collaboration with other disciplines, and mentorship of new faculty colleagues make it imperative that the scope of practice for the academic nurse educator role remains dynamic and continues to evolve. This fourth edition addressing the scope of practice for academic nurse educator roles is evidence of the dynamic evolution of the academic faculty roles.

# References


American Nurses Association. (2015). *Nursing: Scope and standards of practice* (3rd ed.). Author.

American Nurses Association. (2017). American Nurses Association recognition of a nursing specialty, approval of a specialty nursing scope of practice statement, acknowledgment of specialty nursing standards of practice, and affirmation of focused practice competencies. https://www.nursingworld.org/globalassets/docs/ana/3sc-booklet-final-2017-08-17.pdf

Boyer, E. (1990). *Scholarship reconsidered: Priorities of the professoriate*. Carnegie Foundation for the Advancement of Teaching.

Caputi, L., & Engelmann, L. (2004). *Teaching nursing: The art and science*. College of DuPage Press.

Christensen, L. S. (2015). Factors related to success on the Certified Nurse Educator (CNE®) examination [Unpublished doctoral dissertation]. College of St. Mary. https://www.csm.edu/sites/default/files/Christensen_Dissertation_42615.pdf

Christensen, L. S., & Halstead, J. A. (2019). The influence of the core competencies for nurse educators: 2005–2015. In J. A. Halstead (Ed.), *NLN core competencies for nurse educators: A decade of influence* (pp. 1–4). National League for Nursing.

Community Campus Partnerships for Health. (n.d.). *Partnerships that last*. https://www.ccphealth.org

Danna, D. M., Schaubhut, R. M., & Jones, J. R. (2010). From practice to education: Perspectives from three nurse leaders. *Journal of Continuing Nursing Education, 41*(2), 83–87. https://doi.org/10.3928/00220124-20100126-01

Donahue, M. P. (1996). *Nursing, the finest art: An illustrated history* (2nd ed.). Mosby.

Fondiller, S. H. (1999). One hundred years ago: Nursing education at the dawn of the 20th century. *Nursing and Health Care Perspectives, 20*(6), 286–288.

Frenn, M., & Dreifuerst, K. (2019). Summary of research using the NLN core competencies of nurse educators as a framework. In J. A. Halstead (Ed.), *NLN core competencies for nurse educators: A decade of influence* (pp. 5–15). National League for Nursing.

Goldmark, J. (1923). *Nursing and nursing education in the United States* (Report of the Committee for the Study of Nursing Education, and report of a survey by J. Goldmark). Macmillan.

Kalisch, P., & Kalisch, B. (1995). *The advance of American nursing* (3rd ed.). J. B. Lippincott.

Kirkpatrick, J., & Valley, J. (2004). Finding success in the faculty role. In L. Caputi, & L. Englemann (Eds.), *Teaching nursing: The art and science* (pp. 972–989). College of DuPage Press.

Knowles, M., Holton, E., & Swanson, R. (1998). *The adult learner: The definitive classic in adult education and human resource development* (5th ed.). Gulf Professional Publishing.

Kolb, D. A. (1984). *Experiential learning: Experience as a source of learning and development*. Prentice-Hall.

Krathwohl, D. R., Bloom, B. S., & Masia, B. B. (1964). *Taxonomy of educational objectives: The classification of educational goals: Handbook II. Affective domain*. David McKay Company.

National League for Nursing. (2002). *The preparation of nurse educators* [Archived position statement]. https://www.nln.org/docs/default-source/uploadedfiles/about/archived-position-statements/the-preparation-of-nurse-educators-pdf.pdf?sfvrsn=b84cdc0d_0

National League for Nursing. (2005a). *The scope of practice for academic nurse educators*. Author.

National League for Nursing. (2005b). *Transforming nursing education* [Archived position statement]. https://www.nln.org/docs/default-source/uploadedfiles/about/archived-position-statements/transforming052005.pdf?sfvrsn=ac2bdc0d_0

National League for Nursing. (2020). *Hallmarks of excellence*. https://www.nln.org/education/teaching-resources/professional-development-programsteaching-resources/hallmarks-of-excellence-%C2%A9-dffbb05c-7836-6c70-9642-ff00005f0421

National League for Nursing. (2024). *Certified academic clinical nurse educator (CNE®cl) 2024 candidate handbook*. https://www.nln.org/docs/default-source/default-document-library/cnecl-handbook_2024_11.20.2024.pdf?sfvrsn=a5a09c7c_3

National League for Nursing. (n.d.). *Research priorities in nursing education 2024–2027*. https://www.nln.org/education/grants-scholarships/research-priorities-in-nursing-education

Tagliareni, M. E., & Marckx, B. (1997). *Teaching in the community: Preparing nurses for the 21st century*. National League for Nursing.

U.S. Bureau of Labor Statistics. (2025). *Occupational outlook handbook: How to become a licensed practical or licensed vocational nurse*. https://www.bls.gov/ooh/healthcare/licensed-practical-and-licensed-vocational-nurses.htm#tab-4

Appendix A

# *Nursing Education Perspectives* Publications Focused on the Certified Nurse Educator Role

## *NURSING EDUCATION PERSPECTIVES* (NEP) ABSTRACTS

### Defining the Professional Responsibilities of Academic Nurse Educators: The Results of a National Practice Analysis

Tracy A. Ortelli, MS, RN

[*Nursing Education Perspectives*, *27*(5), 242–246, September–October 2006]

#### *Abstract*

In February 2005, the National League for Nursing's Academic Nurse Educator Certification Program and its testing service partner, Applied Measurement Professionals, Inc. (AMP), conducted a study designed to determine the professional practice responsibilities of academic nurse educators. The results of this national practice analysis, reported here, provided the initial information required to ensure the development of a practice-related, content-valid certification examination for academic nurse educators.

### From Committee to Commission: The History of the NLN's Academic Certified Nurse Educator Program

Jan M. Nick, PhD, RNC-OB, CNE, ANEF; Nancy C. Sharts-Hopko, PhD, RN, CNE, FAAN; and Debra Woodard Leners, PhD, RN, PNP, CNE

[*Nursing Education Perspectives*, *34*(5), 298–302, September–October 2013]

#### *Abstract*

**AIM:** To describe the historical events surrounding the development of the National League for Nursing (NLN) Academic Nurse Educator Certification Program (ANECP) and document its transition from a committee to a commission. **BACKGROUND:** During the latter half of the 20th century, certification became a demonstrated standard of excellence in nursing. A few visionaries suggested that nursing education itself was a specialty, but the timing for certification was not right. **METHOD:** The events have been studied through three primary sources: archived minutes, oral interviews, and the authors' eyewitness accounts. **RESULTS:** Growing pains, personnel changes, and the rapid growth from committee to commission occurred during a few short years. While the NLN made sound decisions during the change process by seeking evidence and the guidance of experts and consultants, unexpected challenges occurred. **CONCLUSION:** The tremendous growth of the ANECP in its first years demonstrated that change was clearly desired so long as it was anchored in an evidence-based process focused on quality.

## Preliminary Psychometric Analysis of the Modified Perceived Value of Certification Tool for the Nurse Educator

Tammy Barbé, PhD, RN, CNE

[*Nursing Education Perspectives*, *36*(4), 244–248, July–August 2015]

### Abstract

**AIM:** The purpose of this study was to examine psychometric properties of the Perceived Value of Certification Tool with a focus on nurse educator certification (PVCT®-NE) in a sample of nurse educators. **BACKGROUND:** Greater understanding of faculty perceptions of certification is necessary to facilitate a strong cadre of nursing faculty, but research around nurse educator certification is limited by a lack of reliable and valid instruments to measure such perceptions. **METHOD:** Twenty-four nursing faculty from one university participated in the psychometric study, which involved completion of the PVCT-NE in a web-based survey format. **RESULTS:** Internal consistency reliability was excellent. Cronbach's alpha for the total PVCT-NE was .94 (.93 for the intrinsic subscale and .86 for the extrinsic subscale). A content validity index of .95 was obtained. **CONCLUSION:** There is preliminary evidence that the PVCT-NE is a reliable and valid instrument to measure perceived value of certification in nurse educators.

## Candidates' First-Time Performance on the Certified Nurse Educator Examination

Tracy A. Ortelli, PhD, RN, CNE, ANEF

[*Nursing Education Perspectives*, *37*(4), 189–193, July–August 2016]

### Abstract

**AIM:** This quantitative study examined the first-time pass/fail performance of 2,673 academic nurse educators who took the Certified Nurse Educator (CNE®) examination between September 28, 2005, and September 30, 2011. **BACKGROUND:** This is the first research study designed to analyze candidates' first-time pass/fail performance on the CNE examination. **METHOD:** Descriptive statistics, chi-square test of independence, Pearson's *r* statistic, and binary logistic regression were performed. **RESULTS:** The chi-square test of independence revealed the lack of a statistically significant relationship between study participants' eligibility option and first-time pass/fail performance. Binary logistic regression revealed that a one-year increase in full-time experience resulted in a 1.05 times greater likelihood of passing the CNE examination (OR = 1.05; 95 percent CI 1.03, 1.06; $P = .00$). **CONCLUSION:** This study verifies the need for faculty development and mentoring for nurse educators with less than five years of full-time experience and supports recommendations for doctoral preparation.

## CNE Certification Drive and Exam Results

Michelle M. Byrne, PhD, RN, CNOR, CNE; and Susan Welch, EdD, RN, CCRN, CNE

[*Nursing Education Perspectives*, *37*(4), 221–223, July–August 2016]

### Abstract

The Certified Nurse Educator (CNE®) is the only credential recognizing the advanced practice role of the academic nurse educator. This article provides information regarding a CNE Certification Drive for faculty in one school of nursing. Descriptive findings include pass rates and content-specific averages. An analysis of the relationship between the variables is offered for role (faculty vs. recent graduate), years of teaching, and differences in test scores. Results indicate no significant relationship between role and test results, $\chi^2(1) = 1.11$, $P = .29$, and between years of teaching for those who passed ($M = 10.38$, $SD = 9.81$) versus those who failed ($M = 4.75$, $SD = 6.36$, $t(18) = 1.56$, $P = .14$). Additional research is needed to provide further understanding of variables linked with the CNE exam in multiple schools of nursing.

## What Is the Value of Nurse Educator Certification? A Comparison Study of Certified and Noncertified Nurse Educators

Tammy Barbé, PhD, RN, CNE; and Laura P. Kimble, PhD, RN, FNP-C, FAHA, FAAN

[*Nursing Education Perspectives*, *39*(2), 66–71, March–April 2018]

### Abstract

**AIM:** The purpose of this study was to examine differences in how certified nurse educators and noncertified nurse educators valued nurse educator certification. **BACKGROUND:** No studies have investigated the differences in perceptions of certified and noncertified nurse educators. Understanding these differences may influence how the nursing profession recognizes and promotes excellence within the academic nursing specialty. **METHOD:** Perceived Value of Certification Tool-Nurse Educator and demographic survey were administered via a web-based survey to a national sample of nursing faculty. **RESULTS:** Certified nurse educators valued certification with greater agreement than noncertified nurse educators. Personal accomplishment, personal satisfaction, and validation of knowledge were identified as the greatest rewards of certification. **CONCLUSION:** Nurse educators identified with intrinsic rewards of certification. Despite overall positive perceptions of nurse educator certification, strategies focused on extrinsic rewards may be necessary to increase certification rates. Such strategies may help overcome factors preventing educators from attaining certification.

## Analysis of First-Time Unsuccessful Attempts on the Certified Nurse Educator Examination

John D. Lundeen, EdD, RN, CNE, COI

[*Nursing Education Perspectives*, *39*(2), 72–79, March–April 2018]

### *Abstract*

**AIM:** This retrospective analysis examined first-time unsuccessful attempts on the Certified Nurse Educator (CNE®) examination from September 2005 through September 2011 ($n$ = 390). **BACKGROUND:** There are few studies examining certification within the academic nurse educator role. There is also a lack of evidence to assist nurse educators in understanding those factors that best support success on the CNE exam. **METHOD:** Nonexperimental, descriptive, retrospective correlational design using chi-square test of independence and factorial analyses of variance. **RESULTS:** A statistically significant relationship was found between first-time failure and the highest degree obtained and institutional affiliation on the CNE exam. There was no statistically significant effect on mean scores in any of the six content areas measured by the CNE exam as related to the highest degree or institutional affiliation. **CONCLUSION:** The findings from this study support a previous recommendation for faculty development, experience in the role, and doctoral preparation prior to seeking certification.

## A Factor Analysis of the Perceived Value of Certification Tool for Nurse Educators: Evidence for Construct Validity

Tammy Barbé, PhD, RN, CNE; and Laura P. Kimble, PhD, RN, FNP-C, FAHA, FAAN

[*Nursing Education Perspectives*, *39*(3), E2–E6, May–June 2018]

### *Abstract*

**AIM:** The purpose of this study was to examine construct validity of the Perceived Value of Certification Tool for Nurse Educators (PVCT®-NE). **BACKGROUND:** Preliminary testing of the PVCT-NE demonstrated content validity and strong evidence of internal consistency reliability. Construct validity evidence for the tool is lacking. **METHOD:** Using data from a descriptive study about nurses' perceived value of nurse educator certification, exploratory factor analysis was used to examine whether the factor structure of the PVCT-NE was consistent with the two-factor structure reported for the original PVCT. **RESULTS:** Data ($n$ = 221) were analyzed using principal components analysis to identify factors. The observed two-factor solution and individual item loadings in this sample were consistent with the original PVCT's intrinsic and extrinsic value subscales and accounted for 64 percent of the total instrument variance. **CONCLUSION:** Overall, the PVCT-NE is a valid tool to measure perceived value of certification in nurse educators.

## NLN Core Competencies for Nurse Educators: Are They Present in the Course Descriptions of Academic Nurse Educator Programs?

Ann Fitzgerald, PhD, RN, CNE, FNP-BC; Angela M. McNelis, PhD, RN, FAAN, ANEF, CNE; and Diane M. Billings, EdD, RN, FAAN, ANEF

[*Nursing Education Perspectives*, *41*(1), 4–9, January–February 2020]

### *Abstract*

**AIM:** As an initial approach to determining representation of the NLN Core Competencies for Nurse Educators in Master's of Science in Nursing Education and Post-Master's Certificate programs, the study identified the presence of the competencies in course descriptions. **BACKGROUND:** The competencies are the gold standard to ensure academic nurse educators have the knowledge and skill to teach, assist learners, develop curricula, and implement effective evaluation methods. **METHOD:** A descriptive design that applied web scraping techniques was used to collect data from school web pages, including course descriptions, credit hours, practice information, distance accessibility, and Certified Nurse Educator exam preparation. **RESULTS:** Four competencies were well represented (≥85 percent), and four competencies were poorly represented (<50 percent) in a sample of 529 schools. **CONCLUSION:** Programs should review courses and course descriptions for inclusion of all competency areas that prepare nurse educators and make revisions to address poorly represented competencies.

## A National, Qualitative Study of the Motivators and Outcomes of Nurse Educator Certification

Deborah F. Lindell, DNP, RN, CNE, FAAN, ANEF; Debra Hagler, PhD, RN, ACNS-BC, CNE, CHSE, FAAN, ANEF; and Kathleen Poindexter, PhD, RN, CNE

[*Nursing Education Perspectives*, *41*(6), 327–333, November–December 2020]

### *Abstract*

**AIM:** This qualitative study sought to describe motivators and outcomes of academic nurse educator certification. **BACKGROUND:** Several studies have explored perceptions of the value of nurse educator certification (CNE®). However, there is a gap in understanding motivators and outcomes of certification as a nurse educator. **METHOD:** As part of a larger, web-based, mixed-method study, a national sample of certified and noncertified nursing educator administrators and faculty responded to nine open-ended questions. The inductive content analysis approach was used to identify constructs and themes. **RESULTS:** From an overall sample of 721 participants, three constructs and associated themes emerged. **CONCLUSION:** Motivators for pursuing CNE align with previously reported intrinsic values. Participants seek extrinsic rewards as well. Educator outcomes include enhanced teaching and expanded roles. Student outcomes were less clear. Further study of outcomes of CNE is recommended to promote recognition of academic nursing education as an advanced nursing specialty.

## Using the CNE as an Innovative Strategy to Support Junior Nursing Faculty Transitioning From Clinical Practice

Patricia Kinneary, MS, RN, CNE; and Elizabeth Sutton, MS, RN, CNE

[*Nursing Education Perspectives*, *42*(6), E83–E85, November–December 2021]

### *Abstract*

For new nurse educators, the certified nurse educator credential can be more than a mark of expertise. This article explains how two junior nurse faculty discovered that preparation for certification facilitated the change process from clinician to academic nurse educator. We describe barriers overcome on the path to certification and highlight key factors for attaining success. The important fruits of certification are explored, and recommendations for professional development for new nurse educators are offered.

## Examining the Influence of Academic Nurse Educator Doctoral Degree Preparation on National League for Nursing Core Competency Skill Acquisition

Aaron M. Sebach, PhD, DNP, MBA, AGACNP-BC, FNP-BC, CEN, CPEN, CLNC, CNE, CENcl, SFHM

[*Nursing Education Perspectives*, *42*(5), 272–277, September–October 2021]

### *Abstract*

**AIM:** The purpose of the study was to examine the influence of academic nurse educator doctoral degree preparation on National League for Nursing (NLN) core competency skill acquisition. **BACKGROUND:** Doctor of Nursing Practice (DNP) and Doctor of Philosophy (PhD) graduates frequently seek faculty positions, yet neither degree exclusively prepares graduates for careers in academia. **METHOD:** A descriptive, correlational design was utilized to examine the influence of doctoral degree preparation on NLN core competency skill acquisition. A randomized, nationwide sample ($n$ = 160) of full-time nurse educators teaching in American Association of Colleges of Nursing member schools across the United States completed the Nurse Educator Skill Assessment. **RESULTS:** PhD-prepared educators reported higher NLN core competency skill acquisition scores than DNP-prepared nurse educators. There were statistically significant differences in overall skill acquisition scores between DNP- and

PhD-prepared nurse educators, and for the “use assessment and evaluation” and “engage in scholarship” domains. **CONCLUSION:** These findings provide opportunities for NLN core competency skill acquisition among DNP- and PhD-prepared faculty.

## Passing the Certified Nurse Educator Exam: Innovative Strategies

Sandra A. Basley, MSN, RN-BC, CNE; Debra Erickson-Owens, PhD, RN, CNM, CNE, FACNM, FAAN; Christine McGrane, MS, RN, CNE; Michelle Palmer, MSN, RN, CNE, CNM, FACNM; Mary E. Cloud, MSN, RN, CNE; and Joan R. Dugas, MS, RN, CNE

[*Nursing Education Perspectives*, *42*(6), E79–E80, November–December 2021]

### *Abstract*

Certification in nursing education demonstrates expertise in teaching. The National League for Nursing Certified Nurse Educator credential is a hallmark of excellence. Six academic nurse educators obtained a 100 percent first-time pass rate as a result of a novel cohort model built upon accountability. This article's purpose is to share innovative approaches that can lead to successfully passing the exam.

## NEP FULL TEXT

## From the Editor

### *The Case for Certification and Certification Research*

Joyce Fitzpatrick, Editor

[*Nursing Education Perspectives*, *33*(6), 363, November 2012]

### *Abstract*

> An understanding of the effects of nurse certification on patient outcomes will help nurses and nursing organizations in their quest for professionalism. And outcomes research will be informative to the public and to health care policy makers, who have a keen interest in ways to enhance quality in patient care.

In 2005, the National League for Nursing took a bold step forward to define nursing education as specialty practice. The League implemented the first certification process for nurse educators through the Certified Nurse Educator (CNE) credentialing process to recognize excellence in nursing education. Currently, 3,500 academic educators hold the CNE credential.

With changes to eligibility criteria put into effect in October, the number of CNEs is expected to increase rapidly. But certified nurse educators represent only a small percentage of eligible faculty. In fact, some educators ask: What is the value of certification in nursing education? Why should I become a CNE? The answer is important to our profession.

Certification is an indicator of the specialized knowledge held by an individual. It is not the same as licensure, through which professionals obtain the legal right to practice. We are all familiar with the board certification credentials of physicians, accountants, and psychotherapists. Within nursing as well, there are several specialty areas in which one can become certified, for example, gerontology, critical care, and women's health. In addition, nurses in advanced practice are expected to be nationally certified in their specialty. Although not necessarily a state requirement, national certification is a professional expectation.

In the case of the CNE, the recognition is for the specialized knowledge of nursing education that distinguishes the expert practitioner from others through a formal qualifying and examination process and through the formal recognition of the use of the certification credential, CNE, after one's name. Currently, there are no formal requirements for educator certification within academic institutions. Yet a higher percentage of certified faculty members brings prestige to the school of nursing. The value of certification is that it is acknowledged as prestigious.

As early as 2000, Ann Cary called for research on nurse certification in relation to its effect on nursing practice and patient outcomes. Much of the certification research to date has been focused on benefits to the nursing professional, including both personal and professional benefits. National certification serves as a marker for professional progress for the individual nurse and for the profession.

Yet the need for research, particularly research on patient outcomes, remains of utmost importance, and here is why. An understanding of the effects of nurse certification on patient outcomes will help nurses and nursing organizations in their quest for professionalism. And outcomes research will be informative to the public and to health care policy makers, who have a keen interest in ways to enhance quality in patient care.

As professionals, we have a responsibility to society. We can demonstrate this commitment through research on the benefits of certification.

## President's Message

### *Certification for Nurse Educators: A Mark of Excellence Celebrating Ten Years*

Marsha Howell Adams, NLN President 2013–2015

[*Nursing Education Perspectives*, *36*(4), 207, July–August 2015]

Throughout my time as president of the National League for Nursing and before, I spoke and wrote about the importance of excellence in nursing education. Excellence means not settling for the status quo. It always involves striving to be the best one can be.

One respected illustration of excellence for nurse faculty is the designation certified nurse educator (CNE®). Nurse educators who proudly include CNE in their credentials are recognized for their dedication to and investment in nursing education and nursing, and for their professional accomplishments and commitment to attaining the nurse educator competencies.

In 2005, the NLN published "Transforming Nursing Education," which recommends that "faculty identify themselves as advanced practice nurses *since teaching is an advanced practice role that requires specialized knowledge and advanced education and since certification now exists as a way to recognize expertise in the role*" (www.nln.org/about/position-statements/archived-position-statements, italics added). The Certified Nurse Educator Program, now 10 years old, first received national accreditation in 2009 from the National Commission for Certifying Agencies, renewed in 2014.

The mission of the NLN's Nurse Educator Certification Program is to promote excellence in the advanced specialty role of the academic nurse educator. The goals are to acknowledge the certified nurse educator as an advanced specialty role; recognize the role's knowledge, skills, and abilities required to demonstrate excellence; reinforce the nurse educator competencies; and promote lifelong learning through professional development. As of May 31, 2015, we have 4,887 individuals who have earned the CNE designation. What an accomplishment!

Eligibility requirements for taking the CNE exam have evolved over time and are based on the results of multiple CNE practice analyses. A practice analysis assesses activities undertaken when implementing roles and responsibilities required for a particular professional role. Presently, there are two options whereby an individual can sit for the certification exam. The individual must hold an active RN license and have either: (a) a master's, postmaster's, or doctoral degree with emphasis in nursing education or graduate-level education courses (nine hours) or (b) a master's or doctoral degree in nursing, other than nursing education, and two years of experience in an academic nursing program within the last five years.

I recommend that you visit the NLN website for detailed information about fees and registration: www.nln.org/news/newsroomnln-positiondocuments/archived-position-statements (formerly at www.nln.org/professional-development-programs/Certification-for-Nurse-Educators). For those of you who already hold the CNE designation, the website offers information about recertification. On the website is a link to the *Certified Nurse Educator (CNE) Handbook*, which contains invaluable information and resources to promote success on the exam.

I received my initial CNE designation in 2007 and was recertified in 2012. I found the practice exam to be a huge asset in preparing for the exam because it helped identify gaps in my knowledge and allowed me to focus my preparation time on certain areas. One can also choose to take a live NLN-sponsored review course, given throughout the country on a regular basis and as a preconference option at the NLN Education Summit. In addition, Dr. Linda Caputi has edited the NLN's *Certified Nurse Educator Review*, available for purchase from the NLN Bookstore (nln.lww.com), an essential text for aspiring CNEs and nurse educators across the academic spectrum.

The CNE designation sends a message to our students and our profession about how we value nursing education. I am very proud of my certification as an academic nurse educator and strongly encourage you to join me. In fact, each year at the NLN Education Summit, I, like my peers, carry a handsome red canvas bag signifying that I am a CNE. At the Summit in 2014, red honor cords were introduced for nurse educators to wear during graduation ceremonies. They were a hit.

At the 2015 NLN Education Summit, "A New World of Innovation and Technology," we will hold a special celebration for CNEs to recognize the 10th anniversary of the program. The NLN and its membership are doing great things. I hope you will be there and help us celebrate.

## QUICK READS AND HEADLINES FROM THE NLN

### Preparing for Certification in Nursing Education

Teresa Shellenbarger, DNSc, RN, CNE, ANEF

[*Nursing Education Perspectives*, *29*(6), 330–332, November–December 2008]

Certification in nursing dates back to 1946 for nurse anesthetists (1). Now there are more than 65 certifying organizations, 95 different credentials, and certification in more than 130 nursing specialties (2). Nursing education joined the list of specialties that provide evidence of expertise through certification in fall 2006 with the administration of the first Certified Nurse Educator exam at the NLN Education Summit.

I recently completed the CNE exam and thought it might be helpful to share my experiences. I had been teaching nursing for more than 15 years when I made the decision to pursue certification. I saw certification as potentially helpful with faculty evaluation activities, such as tenure and promotion. Also, since I teach graduate nursing education courses, I hoped to gain some insight into the exam and become a role model for my students. It was particularly important to me to become certified before my students did.

#### *Registering for the Exam*

Having graduated before computer-adaptive NCLEX testing, I decided to take the computerized version of the certification exam, hoping that this experience would help me help my undergraduate students prepare for the NCLEX-RN. While pencil-and-paper testing was available when I registered, it is no longer an option. However, there are a variety of factors to consider when preparing to register for the exam.

First, it is essential to read the *CNE Candidate Handbook* and familiarize yourself with the eligibility requirements, policies and procedures, and fees. (All information and resources pertinent to the NLN Faculty Certification Program are online at www.nln.org/facultycertification/index.htm.) The application takes approximately 10 to 15 minutes to complete. You cannot schedule an examination test date and time until you have completed the registration process and have received a confirmation notice of eligibility.

Once your registration has been processed, you will receive directions for scheduling the exam date and time during a three-month testing window. Consider the timing of the exam and select a convenient date. You will also need to select the test site—one of 120 Applied Measurement Professionals testing centers located throughout the country.

#### *Preparing for the Exam*

The CNE exam was developed based on a practice analysis of nurse educators. This study yielded 119 tasks derived from the *Core Competencies of Nurse Educators with Task Statements* (3). These form the test blueprint, which is available online.

It is important to engage in self-reflection to identify areas of knowledge and any deficits you may have. *The CNE Candidate Handbook* offers sample questions, and a 65-item Self-Assessment Examination that follows the test map and format is available.

This exam gives you the correct answers to questions, along with rationales, and provides for simulation of a computerized exam.

During my personal review, I identified that I had limited experience with online teaching and learning, diverse learners, and psychometrics for multiple-choice exams. Therefore, I focused on this content while reviewing other general areas.

The NLN provides a suggested reference list that may be helpful to review. Many of these classic nursing education sources, used in most graduate nursing education programs, provide the basis for the rationales for the responses. As part of the test preparation, you should also review *The Scope of Practice for Academic Nurse Educators* (4) and consider taking a formal review course. The NLN's biweekly *Faculty Development Bulletin* provides information about certification preparation courses offered throughout the country, and this information is available online at www.nln.org/facultydevelopment/workshopsandconf.htm.

Some faculty find it helpful to work with colleagues to prepare for the exam. Study groups or review sessions with other candidates who are preparing for the test may also be beneficial (5).

## *Test-Taking Reminders*

As you prepare for the exam, keep good test-taking skills in mind. Remember that the people writing the test items are expert nurse educators who know test construction, and all items have been reviewed for content and structure. You will need to rely on your expert knowledge to be successful.

While studying, think prioritization of actions: What do you do first? What is the best response or action? What is the priority? Then, as you take the test, read the entire question, determine what is being asked, read and consider all answers completely, and then select the best response. Sometimes, the response or action that you might use in a real situation is not a choice, so pick the best option from those available.

## *The Day of the Test*

Use a variety of strategies that will help reduce your stress and allow you to arrive early for the exam. If you are traveling to an unfamiliar test site, be sure to have clear directions and a phone number for the test site. You may want to do a preliminary drive to be sure you know where to go and where to park.

Follow the instructions for what you are permitted to bring to the test site, typically two forms of identification and a wallet. Backpacks, bags, and purses are not allowed in the testing area. The exam takes three hours, and there are procedures you need to follow if you must exit for a break, so familiarize yourself with these rules. Wear comfortable clothes, preferably layers that can be removed if necessary.

During the testing session, you will need to complete a series of activities as part of the testing protocol. After providing identification, you will be shown to the testing area, where you will complete a practice exam so that you will know how to proceed through the computer screens. You will be given scratch paper that must be returned at the end of the testing period. During my exam, I did not have a lot of room to write. My testing space was an office cubicle with a traditional computer monitor and keyboard, which I needed to move aside to write my notes.

Make sure to monitor your time and track questions that you want to review. Since you are not penalized for incorrect answers, be sure to complete all questions. Although certain questions are considered experimental and will not count in the final grade, you will not know which these are.

A proctor was not present in the testing room when I took my exam, but all test takers were monitored by video camera. At the start of the exam, the computer was used to take my picture, which remained on the screen during the exam and was printed with the score report.

There are a number of other potential distractions. For example, exams of various lengths are given on the same day, so do not be alarmed if others leave early. When I took the nursing certification exam, I was the only person taking it. And I was seated next to a very nervous young man, retaking a failed exam, who continuously jiggled his leg up and down. It was a challenge to focus on my computer screen.

After you complete the exam, you will need to complete a brief survey about the testing experience. After that is finished, you will submit your scratch paper to the proctor. Unless a new exam is being piloted, you will receive your results immediately. The paper you receive will provide the dates of certification and list specific pass rates for the various sections of the test.

If you are unsuccessful on the exam, you will receive a detailed report of your performance. Take time after the testing session to reflect upon your performance and consider strategies for remediation and retesting. Hopefully, with adequate preparation, you will be successful and will have a reason to celebrate as you join the growing number of CNE professionals.

Certification is good for five years. To renew, you can either take the test again or document professional development activities that relate to at least three competency areas. You will need to keep records of the activity, the date, and the outcome, and complete the certification renewal forms. Select applicants will need to submit supporting documentation as part of the recertification process.

## References

1. Gaberson, K. B., Schroeter, K., Killen, A. R., & Valentine, W. A. (2003). The perceived value of certification by certified peri-operative nurses. *Nursing Outlook, 51*(6), 272–276.
2. Briggs, L. A., Brown, H., Kesten, K., & Heath, J. (2006). Certification: A benchmark for critical care nursing excellence. *Critical Care Nurse, 26*(6), 47–53.
3. Ortelli, T. A. (2006). Defining the professional responsibilities of academic nurse educators: The results of a national practice analysis. *Nursing Education Perspectives, 27*(5), 242–246.
4. National League for Nursing. (2005). *The scope of practice for academic nurse educators*. Author.
5. Kohtz, C., Ferguson, P., Sisk, R., Gowda, C., Smith, J., & Fortson, A. (2008). Quick Reads: The certified nurse educator exam: A plan for success. *Nursing Education Perspectives, 29*(1), 8–9.

# Characteristics of Candidates Who Have Taken the Certified Nurse Educator (CNE) Examination: A Two-Year Review

Tracy Ortelli, MS, RN, CNE

[*Nursing Education Perspectives*, *29*(2), 120–121, March–April 2008]

The National League for Nursing's Certified Nurse Educator (CNE) credential is the only professional credential that recognizes excellence in the advanced specialty role of the academic nurse educator. The CNE examination was initially offered in September 2005 to 206 qualified faculty representing 45 states and the District of Columbia. In the two years in which it has been available, 917 candidates have taken the examination, yielding 773 certified nurse educators. Educators with the CNE credential now represent all 50 states and the District of Columbia.

## *Eligibility Criteria*

The CNE credential requires full-time faculty experience and a master's or doctoral degree in nursing. The two pathways that exist for eligibility are based on educational preparation and faculty experience.

To meet the criteria for Option A, nurse educators must have two years or more of full-time employment in the academic faculty role within the past five years. Further, they must possess a master's or doctoral degree in nursing with either a major emphasis in nursing education or nine or more credit hours of graduate-level education courses.

Nurse educators who possess a master's or doctoral degree in nursing with a major emphasis in a role other than nursing education are eligible for Option B if they have four or more years of full-time employment in the academic faculty role within the past five years. Of the CNE candidates, 64.8 percent met Option A criteria, and 35.2 percent met Option B criteria.

## *Demographic Data*

**Highest Degree Earned.** The highest degree earned by the 917 candidates had nearly even distribution: 34.3 percent of candidates reported holding doctoral degrees, 34.4 percent held master's degrees in nursing with an education focus, and 31.3 percent held master's degrees in nursing with a focus other than nursing education.

To determine if the 917 candidates who took the CNE examination during this two-year period were representative of full-time nurse educators who teach in the United States, demographic data were compared to data described in *Nurse Educators 2006: A Report of the Faculty Census Survey of RN and Graduate Programs* (1). That report notes that nurse educators with doctoral degrees constitute 25.4 percent of the nation's faculty, and those with master's degrees constitute 68.9 percent of faculty. For CNE candidates, the percentages were comparable: 34.3 percent hold doctorates, and 65.7 percent hold master's degrees.

**Primary Teaching Area.** The Certified Nurse Educator examination is available to eligible candidates who teach in all levels of nursing education: practical, diploma, associate degree, baccalaureate, master's, and doctoral nursing programs. Of the candidates who took the CNE examination, 4.5 percent indicated that they taught primarily in practical nursing programs, and 8.8 percent taught in diploma programs. The largest group taught in associate degree programs (39.1 percent), while 36.5 percent taught in baccalaureate programs and 11.0 percent taught primarily at the master's or doctoral level. It is interesting to note that while those who teach primarily in diploma programs represent 3.9 percent of the nation's faculty, they constitute 8.8 percent of the CNE candidate population.

**Years of Full-Time Experience.** The minimum number of years of full-time experience that a CNE candidate may have is two (within the past five years), provided the candidate possesses a master's or doctoral degree in nursing with an education focus. Of those who took the CNE examination, 23.4 percent indicated having two to five years of full-time experience; 39.5 percent reported 6 to 15 years; 25.3 percent reported 16 to 25 years; and 11.8 percent reported more than 26 years of full-time experience.

**Rank.** Nurse educators who hold the rank of instructor constitute the greatest percentage of CNE candidates (29.7 percent) followed by assistant professors (22.8 percent), associate professors (22.1 percent), and professors (16.6 percent). Of the CNE candidates, 9.1 percent indicated they did not hold a rank or title; those who did not indicate rank were typically employed in practical or diploma nursing programs.

**Projected Retirement.** Of the candidates who took the CNE examination during this reporting period, 14.9 percent indicated that they plan to retire within the next five years. Of great concern is the fact that nearly half (46.2 percent) reported that they plan to retire within the next decade and nearly three quarters (71.7 percent) within 15 years.

## *Overall Pass Rate*

The cumulative pass rate for those who took the CNE examination between September 28, 2005 (pilot examination), and September 28, 2007, is 84.1 percent. The consistency of the pass rate over the past two years, during which time it was administered to more than 900 candidates, is one indication of the reliability of the CNE examination.

## *Summary and Future Research*

The CNE examination is offered to a diverse group of qualified, full-time, academic nurse educators who represent the spectrum of nursing program types, academic ranks, years of experience, and educational preparation. Demographic data of CNE candidates reveal that interest in the CNE credential is expressed by nurse educators in all career stages, who teach in all program types. The highest degree earned by candidates was evenly distributed and comparable to national faculty census data.

Candidates were most likely (39.4 percent) to report having six to 15 years of experience. The largest group of CNE candidates held the rank of instructor (29.7 percent) followed by assistant professor (22.8 percent) and associate professor (22.1 percent). Interest in earning the CNE credential may be associated with professional goals of promotion and tenure. Additional research is needed to explore the impact of certification on career advancement as well as the perceived value of certification.

Analysis of candidate performance on each content area of the test blueprint is planned. It is anticipated that these data will provide important information about candidates' knowledge about the Core Competencies of Nurse Educators© (2) as well as the professional development needs of our nation's faculty. The CNE credential, which is the first professional credential designed specifically for nursing faculty, is certain to have a significant influence on nursing education both locally and nationally. The National League for Nursing will closely and carefully evaluate these effects and encourages nurse researchers to investigate this new phenomenon in nursing education.

## *References*

1. National League for Nursing. (2006). *Nurse educators 2006: A report of the faculty census survey of RN and graduate programs*. Author.
2. National League for Nursing. (2005). *Core competencies of nurse educators with task statements*. www.nln.org/facultydevelopment/pdf/corecompetencies.pdf

## The NLN's Certified Nurse Educator Examination (CNE) Program Has Surpassed 5,000 and Gone Global

Larry E. Simmons, PhD, RN, CNE, NEA-BC

[*Nursing Education Perspectives*, *38*(2), 110, March–April 2017]

At the end of 2016, the NLN Academic Nurse Educator Certification (CNE) program is proud to announce that the NLN has certified more than 5,300 nurse educators. This academic nurse certification program, now celebrating its 11th year, establishes nursing education as a specialty area of practice and creates a means for faculty to demonstrate their expertise in this role.

Certification in any field is a mark of professionalism. For academic nurse educators, certification communicates to students, peers, and the academic and health care communities that the highest standards of excellence are being met. By becoming credentialed as a Certified Nurse Educator (CNE), nurse educators serve as leaders and role models in their institutions and throughout the professional nursing community.

The mission of the CNE program is to promote excellence in the advanced specialty role of the academic nurse educator. The goals of the program are as follows:

- To distinguish academic nursing education as a specialty area of practice and an advanced practice role within professional nursing;
- To recognize the academic nurse educator's specialized knowledge, skills, and abilities, and excellence in practice;
- To strengthen the use of core competencies of nurse educator practice; and
- To contribute to nurse educators' professional development.

### *History*

From the program's conception in 2002, when the NLN convened a task group to develop academic nurse educator competencies; to the first pilot examination, administered in 2005 at the NLN Education Summit in Baltimore; to the evolution of the CNE Commission, with a Board of Commissioners; to the first approval of certification by the National Commission for Certifying Agencies (NCCA), a division of the Institute for Credentialing Excellence, in 2008; the program has surpassed expectations for championing the vital role of the academic nurse educator. In 2013, recertification of the program resulted in another five years of NCCA approval.

An exciting recent development has been the opening of the CNE program to global testers. The NLN has affiliated with CGFNS International, Inc. (www.cgfns.org), for validation of eligibility credentials for potential candidates from the international community. As said by NLN president Dr. Anne Bavier, "This partnership has been borne out of long years of collaboration and the complementary strengths that each organization will bring to making the CNE credential available and accessible to nurse educators seeking this leadership recognition in their respective countries." To date, nurse educators in Estonia, the Bahamas, and Germany have successfully passed the CNE examination. Nurse faculty outside the US seeking certification must first apply to CGFNS to have their qualifications evaluated for eligibility. Once approved, faculty may apply to the NLN for authorization to take the CNE examination.

### *Developing a New Examination*

In 2015, the NLN convened a task group to identify competencies for the role of the clinical nurse instructor. These competencies and related task statements were based on current evidence-based literature and developed by educators from both education and practice. In fall 2016, the competencies were presented to the NLN Board of Governors for consideration of creating a new certification examination for clinical nurse educators. The work has now been delegated to the CNE Commission and will proceed through 2017. An NLN publication is also being developed by members of the task group to provide a comprehensive summary of the competencies; it will be available prior to completion of the competency examination. Look for announcements of the examination with a current target date of 2018.

### *Summary*

The NLN is proud and confident that the Academic Nurse Educator Certification program offers quality certification for nurse educators and will continue to meet its goal to advance nurse educator specialty practice. The CNE Board of Commissioners strives to maintain a quality program and pursue new opportunities to enhance the program in the future. More information about the program is available on the NLN website: http://www.nln.org/Certification-for-Nurse-Educators.

## Development of the Certified Nurse Educator Certification Exam: A Spotlight on Competencies, Scoring, and Security

Larry E. Simmons, PhD, RN, CNE, NEA-BC; and Linda Christensen, EdD, JD, RN, CNE

[*Nursing Education Perspectives*, *39*(3), 196, May–June 2018]

To a nurse educator taking a certification exam, the experience may seem similar to that of a student taking an instructor-created exam, but the process is very different, particularly with regard to test development. As we are often asked about the development and scoring of the NLN Certified Nurse Educator certification exam, the following is a brief explanation of how the exam was originally developed, how it remains relevant to current practice, how it is scored, and how security is assured.

## *Test Development*

Certification exams are the end-product of a rigorous test development process. The genesis of certification begins with the identification of the subject matter content/practice competencies and accompanying task statements for the role, which are derived from current literature. The competencies and task statements become the basis for the development of a practice analysis survey by a panel of subject matter experts. Results of the practice analysis are used to develop a test blueprint that outlines and guides test development. To ensure that the test blueprint remains reflective of the current practice of the role, the practice analysis survey is repeated every four to six years.

Subject matter experts write specific test items, each linked to a competency and task statement of the test plan. In addition, each test item must be referenced to current practice literature and conform to the best practices of writing standardized test items. Once the items are developed, they are pilot tested so that the statistical data for the items can be collected and analyzed. Based on item analysis, the test item may be retained "as is" (making it an active exam item suitable for use as a scored item on a test), revised, or deleted. If the item is revised, it must again be piloted before it can be considered active.

## *Data-Driven Scoring*

The NLN certification program uses a minimum of two forms of the certification exam at any one time. Each form must strictly conform to the test blueprint, but the actual test items will vary. Test development committees (TDCs), composed of subject matter experts, are integral in the exam process. The TDC reviews the statistical performance of the individual test items, as well as overall exam performance validity and reliability. This process is data driven. No arbitrary decisions about test items are made during the development and review process.

The passing score for each exam form is set by a method called "cut score setting." The cut score refers to the number of questions that must be answered correctly to pass the exam. The TDC uses a variety of statistical processes in analyzing data to set the cut score, such as the Angoff method or a more general equating method. The final cut score is determined by the TDC in collaboration with experienced psychometricians.

Because there are two forms of the certification exam, each exam's statistics must be examined independently to determine its specific cut score. It is therefore possible that the two exams may have different scores required for passing, with the slightly more difficult exam having a slightly lower passing score.

Test development activities remain a highly secure process. Information about test items is not shared by anyone outside of the test development meetings. Access to the test bank for review is strictly limited to the TDC members and tightly controlled by the agency that provides test administration to candidates.

Periodically, a posttesting candidate requests a review of test items. This is never permitted with a certification exam, as these exams are high-stakes testing for a profession. The security of exams must never be impugned.

Another occasional request is to discard one or more test items from a tester's exam based upon the rationale that there was more than one correct response. Certification items are written so that there is only one correct response that is easily referenced to current literature. Sometimes testers state that certain test items did not reflect their role as a nurse educator. It is important to remember that the certification test is based upon the role competencies and task statements for the role and not on individual practice.

One similarity between a nurse educator taking a certification exam and a student taking an instructor-created classroom exam has to do with preparation. A well-prepared student for a classroom exam will know generally what type of content will be covered and will study accordingly. A well-prepared nurse educator will review the candidate handbook, identify the test plan, and prepare accordingly.

## The Academic Clinical Nurse Educator

Linda Christensen, EdD, JD, RN, CNE; and Larry E. Simmons, PhD, RN, CNE, NEA-BC

[*Nursing Education Perspectives*, *40*(3), 196, May–June 2019]

In the early 2000s, the National League for Nursing (NLN) identified the need to articulate the role of the academic nurse educator. This resulted in the identification of the full scope of the role of the academic nurse educator through the development of evidence-based competencies and related task statements. In early 2015, the idea for articulating the specific role of the academic clinical nurse educator began to take root.

The NLN formed a task group to analyze the literature with the idea of developing role competencies and task statements related to the academic clinical nurse educator role. The task group arrived at consensus on the role and presented the resulting competencies and related task statements to the NLN community for review and feedback. After comments were considered by the task group, the final version of the competencies and task statements was released (September, 2018).

Based on the delineation of the role of the academic clinical nurse educator, a decision was made to move forward with the development of a certification examination. A practice analysis was developed, and academic clinical nurse educators were asked to assist in validation of the task statements associated with the role. The results of the practice analysis provided the basis for the creation of a certification test blueprint. After certification exam test items were developed, two forms of the exam were established, and pilot testing was conducted in the summer/fall of 2018. After passing scores were psychometrically set, the Certified Academic Clinical Nurse Educator (CNE©cl) certification program was officially launched in October 2018.

### *Definition of Practice*

The academic clinical nurse educator may be known by a variety of titles (e.g., clinical faculty, part-time faculty, adjunct faculty, preceptor, clinical instructor). A core definition was developed that would encompass many of the titles being used and clearly delineate the professional role attributes. "The academic nurse educator facilitates the learning of nursing students throughout clinical components of an academic nursing program. The educator is guided...by the faculty of the nursing program and is accountable to the nursing program for providing fair evaluations of learners' performance in meeting expected learning outcomes" (NLN, 2019).

The academic clinical nurse educator submits evaluations of learners' performance that result in academic credit for the clinical learning experience. The academic clinical nurse educator also provides direct supervision of the student learner in the clinical setting. The purpose of the CNEcl certification exam is to validate expertise in the defined role of the academic clinical nurse educator. The goals of the CNEcl certification are as follows:

1. Distinguish academic clinical nursing education as a specialty area of practice.
2. Recognize the academic clinical nurse educator's specialized knowledge, skills, and abilities and excellence in clinical teaching.
3. Strengthen the use of selected core competencies of academic clinical nurse educator practice.
4. Contribute to academic clinical nurse educator clinical practice.

## *Final Thoughts*

The mission of the NLN is to promote excellence in nursing education, to build a strong and diverse nursing workforce, and to advance the health of our nation and the global community. Various products and services of the NLN, such as certification, contribute to meeting the mission. Since the earlier work that established the role of the academic nurse educator, those competencies and task statements have been used as a basis for faculty development, faculty evaluation, curriculum development, and research into the faculty role (Halstead, 2018). The articulation of the academic clinical nurse educator role has the same potential to promote nursing education overall.

Certification in any field stands as achieving a mark of excellence for the certificants. Certifications, particularly in nursing education, are viewed as a mark of distinction and goal attainment for all nursing faculty striving to excel in educational and practice endeavors.

## *References*

Halstead, J. A. (Ed.). (2018). *NLN core competencies for nurse educators: A decade of influence*. National League for Nursing.

National League for Nursing. (2019). *Certified Academic Clinical Nurse Educator (CNE®cl): 2019 candidate handbook*. www.nln.org/Certification-for-Nurse-Educators/cnecl/cne-cl-handbook

# Novice to Expert: Pathways to Nurse Educator Certification

Larry E. Simmons, PhD, RN, CNE, NEA-BC, CGNC, ICE-CPP

[*Nursing Education Perspectives*, *44*(3), 200, May–June 2023]

Since their original release in 2005, the NLN Core Competencies for Nurse Educators and Related Task Statements have provided a framework for curriculum development and revision in graduate nurse educator academic programs, faculty role descriptions, faculty evaluations, and research about nurse educator roles, among other uses (Halstead, 2019). The core competencies and task statements also provided a guide for the development of nurse education certification and the creation of the NLN Certified Nurse Educator (CNE®) program in 2005.

The initial focus of the core competencies was on the role of the academic nurse educator. As our certification program expanded, there was an intentional focus on being inclusive of academic nurse educators at all levels of nursing education, including faculty from diploma, associate degree, and practical nursing programs. After reflection and many development activities, the Certified Academic Clinical Nurse Educator (CNEcl) and Certified Novice Nurse Educator (CNEn) certifications were added to our certification opportunities, creating a framework in line with Benner's novice to expert model of nursing.

## *Certified Nurse Educator*

The competencies were developed for nurse educators practicing in the full scope of the academic role. Since the inception of the CNE®n program, more than 14,000 nurse educators have achieved certification. Many changes in the program were also implemented, including changes in eligibility criteria and, importantly, the opening of the program to the international cadre of nurse educators, resulting in global nurse educator certification. The Board of Commissioners for the Certification Program now includes a Canadian commissioner and a commissioner from Saudi Arabia.

## *Certified Novice Nurse Educator*

In September 2022, the NLN made available a new certification aimed at novice nurse educators (CNE®n), defined as less than three years of nurse educator practice and with competencies leveled to the performance expected of faculty new to nursing education. This certification is a bit different from the others in that it is not renewable, but it opens the door for educators to become confident in the role. We currently have 220 certified novice educators who may wish to continue with CNEcl or CNE certification.

## *Available Resources*

All of these certifications result from the work of task groups that developed the competencies and task statements based on the literature, validated the concepts with member feedback, and performed practice analyses that further validated the concepts, ensuring they are evidence based. The NLN offers useful publications containing in-depth information, including *The Scope of Practice for Academic Nurse Educators* (Christensen & Simmons, 2020) and *Clinical Nurse Educator Competencies: Creating an Evidence-Based Practice for Clinical Nurse Educators* (Shellenbarger, 2019). A new edition of *The Scope of Practice,* to be published in 2023, will provide information on the development of novice educator certification and specific competencies and task statements.

The work of practice analysis committees for each certification program will lead to a new practice analysis every five years, the certification program standard. Each certification has its own handbook, with specific detailed information available at NLN.org as follows: CNE, https://www.nln.org/certification/Certification-for-Nurse-Educators/cne; CNEcl, https://www.nln.org/certification/Certification-for-Nurse-Educators/cne-cl; and CNEn, https://www.nln.org/certification/Certification-for-Nurse-Educators/cne-n.

## *References*

Christensen, L. S., & Simmons, L. E. (2020). *The scope of practice for academic nurse educators and academic clinical nurse educators* (3rd ed.). National League for Nursing.

Halstead, J. A. (2019). *NLN core competencies for nurse educators: A decade of influence*. National League for Nursing.

Shellenbarger, T. (2019). *Clinical nurse educator competencies: Creating an evidence-based practice for clinical nurse educators*. National League for Nursing.

Appendix B

# Acknowledgments

The National League for Nursing (NLN) Core Competencies for Nurse Educators (2005), the Clinical Nurse Educator Competencies (2017), the Novice Nurse Educator Competencies (2021), and the Practical/Vocational Nurse Educator Competencies (2023) were developed by nursing education leaders who had the vision to clearly articulate each of these advanced practice roles of the Academic Nurse Educator. Their work demonstrates the NLN mission to promote excellence in nursing education and build a strong and diverse nursing workforce to advance the health of our nation and the global community.

**The 2005 Academic Nurse Educator Competencies were developed by the NLN Task Group on Nurse Educator Competencies.**

Judith A. Halstead, DNS, RN (Chair)

Wanda Bonnel, PhD, RN

Barbara Chamberlain, MSN, RN, CNS, C, CCRN

Pauline M. Green, PhD, RN

Karolyn R. Hanna, PhD, RN

Carol Heinrich, PhD, RN

Barbara Patterson, PhD, RN

Helen Speziale, EdD, RN

Elizabeth Stokes, EdD, RN

Jane Sumner, PhD, RN

Cesarina Thompson, PhD, RN

Diane M. Tomasic, EdD, RN

Patricia Young, PhD, RN

Mary Anne Rizzolo, EdD, RN, FAAN (NLN Staff Liaison)

**The 2017 Academic Clinical Nurse Educator Competencies were developed by the NLN Task Group on Academic Clinical Nurse Educator Competencies.**

Wanda Bonnel, PhD, APRN, ANEF

Melora D. Ferren, MSN, RN-BC

Erin Killingsworth, PhD, RN, CNE

John D. Lundeen, EdD, RN, CNE, COI

Amber M. Patrick, PhD, RN, CNE, COI

Teresa Shellenbarger, PhD, RN, CNE, ANEF

Linda S. Christensen, EdD, JD, RN, CNE (NLN Staff Liaison)

Larry E. Simmons, PhD, RN, NEA-BC, CNE (NLN Staff Liaison)

**The 2021 Academic Novice Nurse Educator Competencies were developed by the NLN Task Group on Academic Novice Nurse Educator Competencies.**

Rumay Alexander, PhD, RN

Erin Killingsworth, PhD, RN, CNE

Brenda Morris, EdD, RN, CNE

Sharron Schlosser, PhD, RN, CNE

Larry E. Simmons, PhD, RN, CNE (NLN Staff Liaison)

**The 2023 Academic Practical/Vocational Nurse Educator Competencies were developed by the NLN Task Group on Academic Practical/Vocational Nurse Educator Competencies.**

Sarah Billings-Berg, DNP, RN, CNE

Nichelle Bratton, LPN

Irene Coons, PhD, RN, CNE

Jewel Diller, DNP, MSN, RN

Katheryn Doeschot, MSN, RN

Crystal Durham, MSN, RN

Heather Gable, DNP, RN, CNE

Vanessa Lyons, PhD, RN, CNE

Candice Pritchard, MSN-Ed, RN

Benjamin Quintanilla, MSN, RN, NRP

Lagaryion Reed, MSN, RN, CNE

Taylor Reese, MSN, APRN, FNP-BC

Sylvia Silva, RN, BA, DSD

Larry E. Simmons, PhD, RN, CNE, FAAN (NLN Staff Liaison)

MPP1125